Chronic Pain and Addiction

Advances in Psychosomatic Medicine

Vol. 30

Series Editor

T.N. Wise Falls Church, Va.

Editors

G.A. Fava Bologna
I. Fukunishi Tokyo
M.B. Rosenthal Cleveland, Ohio

Chronic Pain and Addiction

Volume Editors

M.R. Clark Baltimore, Md.
G.J. Treisman Baltimore, Md.

10 figures and 14 tables, 2011

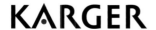

Basel · Freiburg · Paris · London · New York · New Delhi · Bangkok ·
Beijing · Tokyo · Kuala Lumpur · Singapore · Sydney

Advances in Psychosomatic Medicine

Founded 1960 by
F. Deutsch (Cambridge, Mass.)
A. Jores (Hamburg)
B. Stockvis (Leiden)

Continued 1972–1982 by
F. Reichsman (Brooklyn, N.Y.)

Library of Congress Cataloging-in-Publication Data

Chronic pain and addiction / volume editors, M.R. Clark, G.J. Treisman.
    p. ; cm. -- (Advances in psychosomatic medicine, ISSN 0065-3268 ; v. 30)
  Includes bibliographical references and index.
  ISBN 978-3-8055-9725-8 (hard cover : alk. paper) -- ISBN 978-3-8055-9726-5 (e-ISBN)
  1. Chronic pain--Treatment--Complications. 2. Analgesics--Effectiveness. I. Clark, M. R. (Michael R.) II. Treisman, Glenn J., 1956- III. Series: Advances in psychosomatic medicine ; v. 30. 0065-3268
  [DNLM: 1. Chronic Disease. 2. Pain--drug therapy. 3. Analgesics -- therapeutic use. 4. Opioid-Related Disorders--etiology. 5. Substance-Related Disorders--complications. 6. Substance-Related Disorders--etiology. W1 AD81 v.30 2011 / WL 704]
  RB127.C4824 2011
  616' .0472 -- dc22
                                                          2011006954

Bibliographic Indices. This publication is listed in bibliographic services, including Current Contents® and Index Medicus.

© Copyright 2011 by S. Karger AG, P.O. Box, CH–4009 Basel (Switzerland)
www.karger.com
Printed in Switzerland on acid-free paper by Reinhardt Druck, Basel
ISSN 0065–3268
ISBN 978–3–8055–9725–8
e-ISBN 978–3–8055–9726–5

Contents

Clark MR, Treisman GJ (eds): Chronic Pain and Addiction.
Adv Psychosom Med. Basel, Karger, 2011, vol 30, pp 1–7

From Stigmatized Neglect to Active Engagement

Michael R. Clark[a,c] · Glenn J. Treisman[a–d]

Departments of [a]Psychiatry and Behavioral Sciences and [b]Medicine, The Johns Hopkins University
School of Medicine, and [c]Chronic Pain Treatment Program and [d]AIDS Psychiatry Service, The Johns
Hopkins Medical Institutions, Baltimore, Md., USA

Abstract

Chronic pain and substance abuse are common problems. Each entity represents a significant and
independent burden to the patients affected by them, the healthcare system caring for them, and
society at large supporting them. If the two problems occur together, all of these burdens and their
consequences are magnified. Traditional treatments fail a substantial percentage of even the most
straightforward cases. Clearly, new approaches are required for the most complex of cases. Success
is possible only if multiple disciplines provide integrated care that incorporates all of the principles
of substance abuse and chronic pain rehabilitation treatment into one package. While experience
provides the foundation for implementing these programs, research that documents the methods
behind successful outcomes will be needed to sustain support for them.

Copyright © 2011 S. Karger AG, Basel

Chronic pain and substance abuse are independently recognized as complex problems
growing in both scope and severity. Each has its own unique difficulties that contribute to poor outcomes and partial response to treatment. Unfortunately, a substantial
number of patients suffer from both of these devastating problems. These patients
represent a highly stigmatized and uniquely underserved population that would
easily benefit from clinical and research enterprises. Practical and longitudinal expertise is needed for the assessment, formulation and treatment of patients who suffer
with chronic pain and substance dependence disorder. Identifying opportunities and
directions for translational research are important elements in advancing our understanding of these problems and their critically important interrelationships.

In this volume, we have compiled papers related to the topic of chronic pain and
addiction. The epidemic increase in the use of prescription opiates and the increasing
use of opiates for the purpose of euphoria has led to great concern. There has been
an epidemic increase in prescription opiate addiction as well as a dramatic upsurge in

opiate use by adolescents. The increased appreciation of the large number of patients who suffer from chronic pain that diminishes their function is one of the drivers of the increased use of opiates. Unfortunately, many of the medications that are effective at reducing pain are reinforcing and create the potential for addiction.

Refractory Chronic Pain Does Not Equal Addiction

Patients with a poor response to typical treatments for chronic pain are at increased risk of being labeled a 'drug addict' when they request more aggressive pain therapy. Whether they specifically ask for opioid analgesics or not, practitioners will often assume the worst. In patients with known substance use disorder, continuing complaints of pain are routinely regarded simply as drug-seeking behavior that is undermining or counterproductive for their 'recovery' plan. The usual approach to evaluating this complex set of problems devolves to determining whether the patient has a 'real pain' problem or is simply an 'addict'. This dichotomy ends in unsophisticated diagnoses and cookie-cutter treatments.

In contrast, patients with unquestionable chronic pain can and do develop independent substance use disorders that emerge despite the most sincere efforts to seek understandable relief from their pain. Once again, the rush to judgment reflected in the evaluation phase of this problem can lead to the emphasis on only one dimension of the presentation (e.g. substance abuse or pain), which minimizes the other dimension (pain or substance abuse). An essential element in the successful treatment of these patients that present with features of both problems is tolerating the ambiguity that can dominate the initial evaluation and accepting that the question can be resolved with sufficient time in active treatment.

Enhancing Treatment with Integrated Approaches

The common interactions between chronic pain, opioids, and other medical and psychiatric problems including substance use disorders makes treatment-seeking, opioid-dependent patients a critically important subgroup of patients with a compelling need for enhanced evaluation and treatment services [1–3]. Regrettably, patients with chronic pain combined with substance use disorder (especially opioid dependence) remain a stigmatized, maligned and often neglected population [4–6]. Our inability to transmit the public health needs to the individual patient increases the risk for drug-seeking behavior, including self-medication with illicit drugs and the serious hazards associated with this practice.

While the benefits of substance abuse treatment are widely touted, there is little discussion about how routine substance abuse treatment can accommodate the needs of a patient with a comorbid chronic pain syndrome. In addition to patients' inaccurate and underreported use of prescription medications and illicit drugs, the level of difficulty associated with the management of these patients is increased by the infrequent assessment typical of routine chronic pain and drug abuse treatment programs [7, 8]. These problems would be reduced if routine treatment were modified to: (1) incorporate detailed assessments that begin with an extensive history of both prior pain and drug use problems, (2) provide for testing of weekly urine specimens for opioids (prescribed and illicit) and other drugs, and (3) offer ongoing, appropriate positive reinforcements for reporting the use of opioids prescribed by other practitioners to account for the detection of these potentially illicit substances in the urine specimens.

Substance abuse treatment programs should expand their services to address any and all of the comorbidities posing barriers to successful drug rehabilitation. Given the high prevalence and negative impact of chronic pain, new pain management services should be integrated with the drug treatment program and adapted to the patients' need for more intensive treatment. If applied to the problem of chronic pain, a model substance abuse treatment program of integrated stepped care would improve outcomes for patients with both of these devastating types of disorders.

Interdisciplinary Treatment Plans

Interestingly, the treatment of chronic pain in people with substance use disorders remains focused on how to use opioids. There is comparatively little discussion about whether other modalities of therapy might be more effective, safe and appropriate. The assumption that opioids are the first-line therapy for this population further stigmatizes these patients. This position implies that a comprehensive evaluation and treatment plan usually provided to patients without substance use disorders should only be implemented as a last resort in patients with both drug abuse and chronic pain. This recommendation simply accepts that patients with substance use disorder do not have access to high-quality medical care and reinforces the belief that they do not deserve it or that they would reject a priori any alternative to opioid-based treatments.

For example, in the care of this population, there is little discussion of nonopioid medications for the treatment of neuropathic pain problems, interventional approaches to reducing musculoskeletal pain, and active physical therapies to enhance efforts of rehabilitation. Multidisciplinary pain treatment programs have not been incorporated into substance abuse treatment programs, which are not staffed to provide pain evaluation and management. Multidisciplinary pain treatment programs usually seek to avoid patients with clear opioid dependence disorder. The 'hot potato' patients with both problems receive inadequate or no treatment, thereby reinforcing the prophecy that these are 'refractory' cases to be weaned off.

Treating Psychopathology to Optimize Outcomes with Long-Term Opioid Therapy

As a rule, an active substance use disorder is a relative contraindication to chronic opioid therapy. However, opiate therapy can be used successfully if the clinical benefits are deemed to outweigh the risks. A strict treatment structure with therapeutic goals, landmarks to document progress, and contingency plans for noncompliance should be made explicit and agreed upon by the patient and all the providers of healthcare. The first step for the patient is to acknowledge that a problem with medication use exists. The first step for the clinician is to stop the patient's behavior of misusing medications. Then, sustaining factors must be assessed and addressed. These interventions include treating other medical diseases and psychiatric disorders, managing personality vulnerabilities, meeting situational challenges and life stressors, and providing support and understanding. Finally, the habit of taking a medication inappropriately must be extinguished and replaced by more productive, goal-directed activities.

The patient should be engaged in an addiction treatment program that reinforces taking the medication as prescribed and examines the possible reasons for any inappropriate use. Relapse is common and patients with addiction require ongoing monitoring even after the prescription of opioids has ceased. Group therapy is the backbone of treatment for these patients and traditional outpatient drug treatment or 12-step programs can provide a supportive structure for recovery. Relapse prevention should rely on family members or sponsors to assist the patient in getting prompt attention before further deterioration occurs. If relapse is detected, the precipitating incident should be examined and strategies to avoid another relapse should be implemented. Although the misuse of medications is unacceptable, neither total abstinence nor complete compliance is always possible. Restoration of function should be the primary treatment goal and may improve with adequate, judicious and appropriate use of medications, even if setbacks occur [9].

A comprehensive formulation is necessary for the determination of why long-term opioid therapy is not working to control a patient's pain and causing deterioration in function. Approaching patients by investigating the different perspectives of acquired diseases, inherent vulnerabilities, disruptive choices and unfulfilling encounters focuses the physician on treatable causes of disability instead of blaming the patients or their opioids for a lack of rehabilitative progress.

Future Research

There is a growing consensus that the prevalence of cooccurring chronic pain and substance use disorders is high and presents a significant burden to the healthcare system and society. Treatment approaches that target either one of these problems run the risk of ignoring the other and compromising the overall care and prognosis of these patients. Cartesian dualism in any form is an inadequate model for the assessment, formulation and treatment of patients. These patients cannot be clearly understood from an 'either/or' perspective. Attributions of all of the patient's symptoms to either chronic pain or substance use disorder often fail to appreciate the complex relationships between these problems and other relevant factors. In combination with limited access to integrated treatment programs and settings, the outcome for many of these patients remains grim. Future research is necessary to help guide progress. Studies that provide a more comprehensive evaluation of both problems and prospective characterization of chronic pain problems in opioid-dependent patients seeking outpatient methadone treatment would be most helpful. Just as important, interventions for chronic pain to improve the response to drug abuse treatment are needed.

These new efforts should expand existing expertise in the assessment of psychiatric comorbidity and integrated treatment delivery models to the domain of chronic pain, which is clearly an underdiagnosed and poorly treated medical and psychiatric problem in patients with substance use disorders. Increasing the utilization of nonopioid medications typically used to treat chronic neuropathic pain conditions, such as antidepressants and anticonvulsants, which are underutilized in general medical care and rarely prescribed to patients with substance use disorders, should become a priority [5]. Improving access to comprehensive pain treatment programs would offer more hope to patients with chronic pain and substance abuse than continuing to advocate the use of unimodal therapies like long-term opioid agonists [10, 11].

Implementing and evaluating the principles of rehabilitation utilized by multidisciplinary pain centers and selected substance abuse treatment programs would deepen our understanding of the associations between chronic pain and response to highly structured adaptive drug abuse treatment settings. These data would improve outcomes and provide a strengthened empirical foundation for the design and implementation of clinical trials to reduce the suffering and impairment associated with chronic pain in people with chronic and severe opioid dependence disorder. The results would likely generalize to other populations of patients with chronic pain to improve our understanding of the risks of treatment with opioids and, hopefully, prevent the development of opioid dependence disorders in at least some of these high-risk individuals.

Conclusions

The topic of chronic pain and addiction is divisive, with proponents of aggressive opiate use arguing that addiction in patients with chronic pain syndromes is relatively rare, while those who push for more conservative use argue that opiates cause disorder in many patients and are relatively ineffective against chronic pain over time. There is some discord among the authors in this volume, in part driven by the focus of their work, but several points of agreement come through. From the consensus here, several points of agreement emerge.

First, the simplistic concept of addiction as physical dependence and that addiction is mostly a matter of withdrawal is inadequate. A clearer definition of what addiction is comprised of and a better understanding of the factors that lead to disordering use of pain medications is crucial. The behavioral perspective as well as a basic physiological understanding of addition is critical for developing better models.

Second, chronic pain is physiologically diverse and complicated. The extreme capacity for adaptation of pain systems including integration, regulation and crosstalk at nearly every level of the nervous system argues for the importance of nociceptive senses for survival and function. The development of better models for understanding and preventing chronic pain is crucial for understanding treatment alternatives for patients suffering from chronic pain. Chronic pain syndromes caused by nerve dysfunction such as neuropathy overlap with those caused by denervation, central upregulation syndromes and sympathetic pain syndromes. Clearer models are needed to help determine effective treatment alternatives.

Third, the development of more selective pain therapies is of utmost importance. Diverse circuitry and neurotransmitter systems are involved in chronic pain, and the work on ketamine, cannabinoids, selective opiates and other novel targets such as N-methyl-D-aspartic acid receptors is very exciting. How these alternatives will impact potential addictive behavior is a key area of investigation.

Fourth, better tools for clinicians to predict and prevent the development of addictive and disordering drug use are needed. The development of addictive and disordering behaviors does not mitigate the ongoing pain that patients experience. Effective ways to treat chronic pain in patients with addictions, and to improve function and restore quality of life for patients requires an interdisciplinary understanding and treatment. The contributions of medical pathology, physical limitations, depression, personality, family dynamics, patients' self-concept, and social and cultural factors must be assessed and included when trying to treat comorbid pain and addiction.

Lastly, the high prevalence of chronic pain syndromes has been explored in patients seeking treatment for drug abuse only recently. The presence of chronic pain increases the risk of poor response to substance abuse treatment along with an increased likelihood of multiple comorbidities that further add to the negative impact experienced by patients with substance dependence disorders. Substance abuse treatment programs that offer integrated medical and psychiatric care for these comorbidities would improve outcomes. Stepped-care treatment approaches offer the best substance abuse treatment by tailoring the level of care to the needs of the individual patient.

In summary, this volume was developed to review the fundamental issues that underlie this complex and contentious area. We wish to thank the authors for their contributions, hard work, patience and collegiality. We feel privileged that our friends and colleagues were willing to contribute their work to our efforts. We sincerely hope the readers of this volume will find it valuable for their understanding of these patients and for their own work on helping their patients back to functional and healthy lives.

References

1 Cohen MJ, Jasser S, Herron PD, Margolis CG: Ethical perspectives: opioid treatment of chronic pain in the context of addiction. Clin J Pain 2002; 18(suppl):S99–S107.

2 Drug Enforcement Administration: A joint statement from 21 health organizations and the Drug Enforcement Administration. Promoting pain relief and preventing abuse of pain medications: a critical balancing act. J Pain Symptom Manage 2002;24:147.

3 Nicholson B: Responsible prescribing of opioids for the management of chronic pain. Drugs 2003;63: 17–32.

4 Gilson AM, Joranson DE: US policies relevant to the prescribing of opioid analgesics for the treatment of pain in patients with addictive disease. Clin J Pain 2002;18(suppl):S91–S98.

5 Rosenblum A, Joseph H, Fong C, Kipnis S, Cleland C, Portenoy RK: Prevalence and characteristics of chronic pain among chemically dependent patients in methadone maintenance and residential treatment facilities. JAMA 2003;289:2370–2378.

6 Peles E, Schreiber S, Gordon J, Adelson M: Significantly higher methadone dose for methadone maintenance treatment (MMT) patients with chronic pain. Pain 2005;113:340–346.

7 Ready LB, Sarkis E, Turner JA: Self-reported vs actual use of medications in chronic pain patients. Pain 1982;12:285–294.

8 Fishbain DA, Cutler RB, Rosomoff HL, Rosomoff RS: Validity of self-reported drug use in chronic pain patients. Clin J Pain 1999;15:184–191.

9 Currie SR, Hodgins DC, Crabtree A, Jacobi J, Armstrong SJ: Outcome from integrated pain management treatment for recovering substance abusers. Pain 2003;4:91–100.

10 Scimeca MM, Savage SR, Portenoy R, Lowinson J: Treatment of pain in methadone-maintained patients. Mt Sinai J Med 2000;67:412–422.

11 Ziegler PP: Addiction and the treatment of pain. Subst Use Misuse 2005;40:1945–1954, 2043–2048.

Michael R. Clark, MD, MPH
Department of Psychiatry and Behavioral Sciences
Osler 320, The Johns Hopkins Hospital, 600 North Wolfe Street
Baltimore, MD 21287-5371 (USA)
Tel. +1 410 955 2126, E-Mail mclark9@jhmi.edu

Clark MR, Treisman GJ (eds): Chronic Pain and Addiction.
Adv Psychosom Med. Basel, Karger, 2011, vol 30, pp 8–21

A Behaviorist Perspective

Glenn J. Treisman[a–d] · Michael R. Clark[a,d]

Departments of [a]Psychiatry and Behavioral Sciences and [b]Medicine, The Johns Hopkins University School of Medicine, and [c]AIDS Psychiatry Service and [d]Chronic Pain Treatment Program, The Johns Hopkins Medical Institutions, Baltimore, Md., USA

Abstract

Chronic pain is a sensory experience that produces suffering and functional impairment and is the result of both sensory input as well as secondary adaptation of the nervous system. The sensitization of the nervous system to pain is influenced by physical activity (or inactivity) and medication exposure. Medication taking and physical activity are behaviors that are increased or decreased by positive and negative reinforcement. Patients often have comorbid psychiatric conditions at presentation, including addictions, mood disorders, personality vulnerabilities and life circumstances that amplify their disability and impede their recovery. Behavioral conditioning contributes to chronic pain disorders in the form of both classical (Pavlov) and operant (Skinner) conditioning that increases the experience of pain, the liability to ongoing injury, the central amplification of pain, the use of reinforcing medications such as opiates and benzodiazepines, and behaviors associated with disability. The term 'abnormal illness behavior' has been used to describe behaviors that are associated with illness but are not explained physiologically. Behavioral conditioning often amplifies these abnormal behaviors in patients with chronic pain. Addiction can also be seen as a behavior that is reinforced and conditioned. The same factors that amplify abnormal illness behaviors also increase the liability to addiction. Psychiatric comorbidities also complicate and amplify abnormal illness behaviors and addictive behaviors and further contribute to the disability of chronic pain patients. Model interventions that reinforce healthy behaviors and extinguish illness behaviors are effective in patients with addictions and chronic pain. Maladaptive behaviors including addictive behaviors can be used as targets for classical and operant conditioning techniques, and these techniques are demonstrably effective in patients with chronic pain and addictions.   Copyright © 2011 S. Karger AG, Basel

Despite the strides made in the area of disease treatment over the centuries, the field of medicine has struggled with the issues of chronic pain throughout its history. The very goal of medical care has been debated with function, quality of life, longevity and comfort all vying for primacy. In advanced cancer cases, the goals of longevity and function are often beyond our current capabilities, and therefore quality of life and comfort become the targets. At the other end of the spectrum are patients with psychological distress underlying their chronic noncancer pain, and they need ongoing orientation toward function and longevity. The current conundrum of opiate use in chronic pain is mostly driven by an inadequate understanding of the differences between chronic pain and acute pain, cultural issues about patient autonomy and entitlement to comfort, and the effort to create efficiency in medical care at the cost of a comprehensive formulation of patients as individuals with complex physical and psychological pathologies that need individualized treatment plans.

For the purposes of this discussion, we will divide pain into acute pain, as defined by a noxious sensation directly provoked by tissue injury or damage, and chronic pain, as defined by a noxious sensation occurring after the resolution of tissue injury. This leaves a group of patients, those with ongoing chronic tissue injury (e.g. rheumatoid arthritis or ischemia), falling into the acute pain group despite the chronic nature of their illness. Nerve damage such as neuropathy and central upregulation syndromes will be considered together for the moment, although experimental models distinguishing them have been developed.

Pain has two well-described components, a sensory element that is sometimes described as nociceptive, and an emotional component of distress. At lower doses, opiates preferentially relieve the emotional element. Patients will say they can still feel the pain but they find it less objectionable. Unfortunately, opiates produce tolerance to this element of their action, and the distress returns with continued opiate use over time. Patients who are disordered by chronic pain do not differ from patients with nondisordering pain with respect to the type of pain, its severity or its location. Instead, increasing emotional distress and disability lead to an increasing emphasis on trying to relieve pain rather than function despite it.

Chronic pain is influenced by a variety of factors. We will discuss depression, personality, life experiences and behavioral conditioning, with a central focus on behavioral conditioning and reinforcement.

Behavior and Chronic Pain

William Fordyce may be seen as the father of behaviorist approaches to chronic pain and rehabilitation. He noticed that patients who did well in rehabilitation differed from those who did poorly in what they did rather than the severity of their illness and its resultant pathology. He read the work of B.F. Skinner and decided to try to focus on using behavioral techniques to enhance the rehabilitative efforts of patients. He coined the term 'pain behavior', and his work revealed that getting patients to change behavior to increase function in rehabilitation resulted in better outcomes [1].

Issy Pilowski, a contemporary of Fordyce, did the ground-breaking work on abnormal illness behaviors that focused on the fact that patients often seek the 'sick role' despite a lack of physiological findings to support the degree of dysfunction they manifest. He additionally described that they do not share the goal of rehabilitation and improving function with their doctor, but rather seem committed to continuing in the sick role and refuse the responsibilities inherent in rehabilitative treatment. They believe that they 'can't' do things that they do not feel emotionally inclined to do. As a result, they often say that they 'can't' attend physical therapy, engage in psychological treatments or tolerate medications that do not immediately relieve their discomfort. They usually end up on treatments that have no pain efficacy (such as benzodiazepines) or have lost effectiveness (opiates) but do not continue treatments (even those that have been shown to be helpful to them) that provide chronic diminution of the sensory complaints that underlie their disorder of chronic pain [2].

The behavioral approach to patients with chronic pain helps produce a coherent understanding of how patients develop maladaptive behaviors, and is the basis for analyzing factors that delay recovery and amplify dysfunction. The behavioral approach also provides a framework for a treatment plan that focuses on rehabilitation, function, quality of life and healthy behavior that does not imply that patients are 'feigning' their illness.

Behavior is a goal-directed activity that either increases with reinforcement or decreases with a lack of reinforcement. In the early 1900s, Pavlov described conditioning as the pairing of unrelated stimuli (such as the ringing of a bell) with the presence of stimuli usually associated with a particular behavior (the presence of food is the stimulus for the behavior of salivation). Clinical examples of 'classical' or 'pavlovian' conditioning include the gradual development of nausea in cancer patients when arriving at the cancer center even before the administration of chemotherapy [3]. Many patients spontaneously vomit on arrival at the clinic, even on visits that take place after chemotherapy has concluded. A similar phenomenon is described by opiate users who have experienced 'cold turkey' opiate withdrawal in a particular environment and later experience withdrawal symptoms when exposed to that environment even after complete discontinuation of opiates. Conditioned withdrawal can easily be produced in experimental animals using this paradigm [4].

B.F. Skinner described operant conditioning as the shaping of behavior using positive or negative responses to the behavior [5]. He described four types of operant reinforcement, as shown in table 1: positive reinforcement, where a behavior results in the delivery of something that is rewarding; negative reinforcement, where the behavior results in the removal of something unpleasant; punishment, where the behavior results in the delivery of something unpleasant, and extinction, where the behavior results in the removal or lack of delivery of something rewarding.

It is common to see medical applications of operant conditioning at work in patients. Opiates can be used in laboratory settings to shape behavior and reward animals (see the discussion by Gardner [this vol., pp. 22–60]). Animals learn to perform behaviors for opiate rewards, such as pulling levers (primates), pecking keys (birds) and pressing bars (rodents). In experiments, animals can be taught to work to get access to opiates, and then be asked to tolerate increasingly adverse stimuli (electric shocks/food deprivation) to get access to opiates. Opiates have powerful rewarding

Table 1. Summary of operant conditioning (as described by B.F. Skinner)

		Stimulus quality	
		positive	negative
Stimulus when behavior occurs	deliver	positive reinforcement (behavior increases)	punishment (behavior decreases)
	withdraw	extinction (behavior decreases)	negative reinforcement (behavior increases)

Four cells of operant conditioning: positive reinforcement, where a behavior results in the delivery of something that is rewarding (increases the behavior); negative reinforcement, where the behavior results in the removal of something unpleasant (increases the behavior); punishment, where the behavior results in the delivery of something unpleasant (decreases the behavior), and extinction, where the behavior results in the removal or lack of delivery of something rewarding (decreases the behavior).

effects in humans, and therefore behaviors associated with the administration of opiates increase in frequency and intensity if they consistently result in opiate rewards. Clinicians have been shown to prescribe opiates in response to nonverbal pain behaviors, and opiates are often given in response to these behaviors in hospital settings [6]. Physicians also are more likely to prescribe opiates in response to the emotional elements of pain, so that distress is reinforced and encouraged to increase over time.

A separate question is whether patients can actually be conditioned to experience pain. It is clear that circling a number on a visual analog scale is a behavior that is affected by opiates, such that higher scores occur in patients who get opiates simply as a response to higher scores. Nociceptive transmission is enhanced by opiates [7]. Not only are the behaviors related to pain increased by opiate rewards, the pain itself can probably be increased by contingent administration of opiates.

Positive reinforcement by opiates is easy to model experimentally, but negative reinforcement also occurs. Both pain and opiate withdrawal are aversive experiences, and the administration of opiates relieves the adverse experience, leading to another negative reinforcement. Negative reinforcement is equally important in directing behavior in patients with chronic pain. A specific example is the patient who described his unpleasant marriage, detested job and difficult life. His only real pleasure was playing softball. After an ankle sprain, he went to the emergency room (ER), where he received an injection of meperidine and experienced the sudden relief of pain. He was also given a note to miss work, and his wife was told that he should be allowed to rest. He described how he remembered the note for work and the meperidine when he sprained his ankle the second time, and how he did not really 'need' to go to the ER but went anyway and had a similar experience. He described how after those two experiences, he began to visit ER with increasing frequency to obtain relief from his

Table 2. Examples of reinforcers of abnormal illness behavior

Positive reinforcers
Opiates and benzodiazepines
Disability payments
Attention from spouses, family, doctors, lawyers
Ability to express prohibited feelings
Possibility of 'lump sum' payments
Negative reinforcers
Relief from requirements of work and related stress
Relief from expectations and criticism by others
Relief from depression and low self-esteem/negative self-worth
Relief from psychological discomfort and distress
Relief from pain and physical discomfort

distress, including opiates, pleasant attention from attractive nurses, and notes relieving him from responsibilities until he had 'lost everything'. When he presented for evaluation, he had lost his job and his marriage and was in deep financial difficulty, facing homelessness, and dependent on his parents for support.

The illness behaviors of patients with chronic pain are reinforced by numerous elements of their everyday existence. Common reinforcers are shown in table 2. Although clinicians may react to the behavior as if it were a conscious effort by the patient to deceive them, patients are often unaware of the factors that condition them to behave in particular ways, and feel that they 'can't help it'. Although the behavior is deliberate and designed to manipulate, it has become reflexive and feels automatic. Cancer patients can be told the IV fluid that they get is normal saline, but if they have been conditioned to vomit from repeated exposure to chemotherapy, they are unable to prevent the vomiting from occurring.

Unfortunately, the medical system has produced a variety of factors that particularly affect vulnerable patients. David Edwin has described 'abnormal doctoring behavior' in much the same way Izzy Pilowski described abnormal illness behavior. Dr. Edwin describes how patients and other factors inadvertently condition doctors to behave in maladaptive ways. Doctors are as susceptible to conditioning as any other organism. A variety of external forces are imposed on medical practice that may condition doctors to deliver care in particular ways. Doctors may be conditioned to reward dependent and disability-related behaviors inadvertently. As an example, patients who are admitted to the hospital without insurance receive expedited medical coverage if they are disabled and receive disability benefits. Well-meaning doctors recognize that disability status means resources. Hospitals actively encourage doctors and social workers to expedite disability paperwork for these patients, and there are lawyers who specialize in obtaining disability benefits for patients. Although patients 'can' always go back to work, they are less likely to do so once they start to receive payment for being ill.

Perhaps the most striking example of this is the development of the visual analog pain scale and the imposed requirement to use it in medical practice. Over the past several decades, a number of studies have been published showing that doctors have been reluctant to prescribe opiates to terminal cancer patients because of a reflexive resistance to causing opiate dependence. As was accurately pointed out in these studies, cancer pain was undertreated without a good rationale. Concerns about the undertreatment of pain prompted numerous studies and interventions directed at better assessment and pain control. These were soon directed at a variety of pain situations, and standards were described for assessment and control of pain in general. Unfortunately, a fad developed around the treatment of pain with little distinction between acute postsurgical pain, pain associated with cancer, and chronic nonmalignant pain conditions. Pain was made a 'vital sign' as a result of political rather than scientific concern. Getting on the bandwagon somewhat late in the game, the Joint Commission on Accreditation of Healthcare Organizations required 'all' patients seen in hospital settings to have an evaluation of pain at every visit, and required a definition of 'pain emergencies' and a response strategy for them. While this strategy may reduce pain, it might also reduce function, and some types of pain need chronic rehabilitation and physical therapy rather than a focus on suppression. 'Vulnerable' patients are conditioned by this paradigm to seek narcotics, and doctors are conditioned to prescribe them. We have had many patients tell us that their pain score is above an '8' and that they are therefore entitled to receive narcotics as an emergency. As a striking example, one patient said: 'I prefer Demerol but I know that you doctors have problems with abuse so I will have 8 mg of i.v. Dilaudid and 50 mg of Phenergan. You don't have to look it up, that's the right dose.' A massive increase in opiate use under these conditions is no surprise.

It is also no surprise that the doctors are now being blamed for the problem. While we can describe the pressures that resulted in increased opiate use for chronic nonmalignant pain with few data to support its effectiveness for most of the types of chronic pain, this does not excuse the practice. Doctors allowed themselves to be directed to do this, sometimes to the detriment of their patients. The doctor-patient relationship evolved to protect patients from fads in medicine and outside influences that are detrimental to patients. The current systematized corruption of this relationship by our consumerist society, financial motives to increase the profitability of medicine, and the antipaternalist political climate in medicine must be resisted by physicians. Regardless of the political climate of the moment, doctors will be held accountable for their actions if they harm patients, and the current fad of seeing patients as 'customers' to be 'satisfied' is clearly harming vulnerable patients who cannot protect themselves. Table 3 shows some other examples of these trends. Because addiction is essentially a biologically driven, conditioned behavior, the

Table 3. Behavioral reinforcement of maladaptive behaviors in doctors and patients

Normal doctor behavior being distorted	Abnormal doctor behavior	Reinforcer of abnormal doctor behavior	Maladaptive patient behavior reinforced
Diagnosis-directed treatment	Symptom-directed treatment	Short visits; financial efficiency	Focus on complaints
Rational strategic therapy for rehabilitation	Allowing patient to chose medications (opiates and benzodiazepines)	Patient 'autonomy'; patient 'satisfaction' and fear of complaints	Increasing medication dependence; using medication to cope
A single coordinating primary physician who communicates with consultants and controls treatment	Allowing patients to receive care from multiple non-communicating sources	No reimbursement for time spent communicating; multiple barriers to physician communication (HIPAA)	Patients increasingly choosing doctors directed at comfort rather than rehabilitation; 'splitting' of clinicians
Thorough formulation and individualized treatment planning	Using algorithms for treatment	Fear of criticism; increasing bureaucratic regulation of medical care with guidelines becoming 'recipes'	Identification of themselves as a 'patient' and increasing the sick role
Comprehensive assessment of the type of pain quality, location, mitigating and exacerbating features	Pain as a vital sign and linear assessment of pain severity	Increasing bureaucratic regulation of efficient medical care with required 'measures' that oversimplify cases	Amplification of pain complaints and escalating need for narcotics to meet the target number on a visual analog scale

HIPAA = Health Insurance Portability and Accountability Act.

above elements of pain treatment clearly predispose vulnerable patients to develop addictive behaviors.

A Behavioral Model of Addiction

The difficulty in defining addiction is that it is a process that evolves rather than a discrete change. The discussion of dependence, reinforcement, tolerance and pseudo-addiction in other papers in this volume and in the literature attempt to make black-

and-white distinctions in opiate use and addictive behavior. Opiates are dependence producing and reinforcing, and yet many patients are not 'disordered' by them. An important point to include here is that dependence does not always produce addiction. The majority of patients treated for pain with opiates who become physically dependent on opiates successfully withdraw from opiates as they get better. We define addiction as the disordered behavior produced by the increased seeking and use of a substance despite mounting negative consequences. This is a simple behavioral definition and leaves something to be desired by those who want a clear 'category' for when a patient is an addict, but accounts for much of the difficulty in deciding how to manage behavioral irregularities in patients. Addictive behaviors such as deception, intoxication, personality deterioration and self-destructive actions all develop over time with continued drug administration and are reinforced by the drug being used. When describing addictions, it is important to note that these same behaviors can be conditioned to occur in animals, and that it is the drugs that are addictive, and not the patient who is somehow a latent addict. This is not to deny that patients (and animals) clearly vary in their vulnerability to addictive behavior (as we will discuss below) as many elements of vulnerability (genetic, temperamental, social, environmental and psychiatric comorbidity) have been demonstrated by valid research.

The behavioral model we use is conceptualized in figure 1 [8]. Many behaviors are conditioned by external factors as described above, but a subset of behaviors also involve an internal reward 'loop', such as eating, sleeping and sexual activity, linked directly to the reward circuitry of the brain, which generates appetites or drive states. Patients describe a 'hunger' for these behaviors. All motivated behaviors (eating, sleeping, sex) are driven by visceral and neuroendocrine elements. In the case of addiction, most substances of abuse have a strong effect on the mesolimbic dopaminergic system of the brain. Additionally, opiate systems in the brain are an independent but linked reward system that directly activates this cycle. The mesolimbic structures are among the most primitive structures of the brain and affect behavior at its most fundamental level. When animals are allowed to medicate themselves with substances of abuse, their behavior closely mimics that of humans. The driven, out-of-control feeling that addicts describe is mediated by this biological mechanism.

At the top of figure 1 is the external reinforcement, but below we show the cycle of internal reinforcement that is associated with the positive feedback cycle of motivated behaviors. This cycle serves the purpose of amplifying behavior. As children learn, they eat, get an internal sense of reward, and gradually develop increasing interest in eating. While this behavior can become out of control, it is tightly regulated as an evolutionary safeguard, and there is a point at which appetite is shut off and someone has 'had enough'. The salience of behavior changes as well. Before eating, reading the menu is interesting, and one might even read about food that one would never really want to eat, but after dinner the menu has no salience, and reading it might even be faintly sickening. The 'turning off' or inhibition of the drive to eat is activated after the behavior of eating. When the turning off is faulty, eating behavior will go awry.

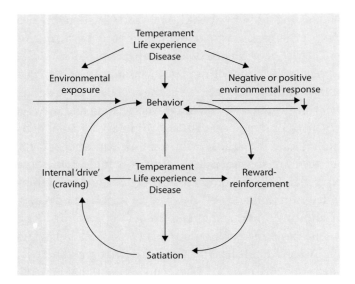

Fig. 1. Behavioral amplification cycle for normal and addictive behaviors. The diagram illustrates how behaviors are conditioned by external factors in the top part of the figure. Positive and negative feedback 'condition' an increase or decrease in behaviors. The lower part of the diagram illustrates how certain behaviors are 'amplified' by the loop shown to dramatically increase the likelihood of the behavior and to prevent aversive experiences from extinguishing it. The cycle can be modified by the psychiatric comorbidities shown as well as other factors.

Positive feedback loops are inherently dangerous in biology. An important teleological question is why a positive feedback cycle that has the ability to get so out of control should be present. Behaviors associated with survival need to be amplified at certain times. The 'internal rewards' described above are only present for these important survival behaviors. Although aversive experiences such as food poisoning can condition people not to eat anything even remotely like the food that made them sick, and can result in a lifetime dislike of a particular food, feeding itself is necessary for survival. The amplification cycle insures that people will eventually eat again, and that behaviors needed for survival will continue to occur, even if at a reduced frequency for some time. The power of this loop to condition behavior so that it will overcome even intensely aversive experiences is amply demonstrated by the resilience of behaviors involving eating, sleeping, drinking and sexual activity.

The central issue for drug users is that unlike feeding, sleeping and sexual behaviors, addictive compounds were not present in the environment during the millions of years that this cycle took to evolve, and therefore the intrinsic 'turn-off' mechanism for these survival behaviors is not present for drug use. This makes the susceptibility to substance use disorders stronger and more dependent on exposure than disorders of other motivated behaviors.

Treisman · Clark

Given this description, why doesn't everyone get addicted? The cycle is inhibited and shaped by many factors. Biological factors such as genetics and underlying features of temperament such as introversion are discussed below. Social factors that have been shown to provide protection against addiction include close family and social structures, connections to others in the form of marital and social relationships, commitments to career and occupational life and internalized structures such as religion and moral stance. All of these have been shown to protect individuals from addiction and act as a 'brake' on the cycle shown above. To some extent they immunize people against drug use disorders. In fact, those that become dependent on substances and develop disorders associated with substance use are often in transitions during which the usual structure of life breaks down. Loss of jobs and breakup of relationships are common concomitants of drug use getting out of control. The patient may always have used a little too much alcohol, but now has lost his job and therefore does not need to get up in the morning. The student leaving home for college has no early classes and dramatically less supervision. The young person with a service job at McDonald's loses little if he is fired there because he can get hired at Burger King. A person with a difficult-to-obtain position risks more and loses more if he is fired, and therefore is relatively more protected. Our patient who got addicted to Demerol and ER visits was 'vulnerable'. He was poorly protected by his circumstances and fell into addictive behaviors easily and rapidly. Many other patients are resilient, and develop their addictions very slowly and after years of successful treatment with opiates.

Psychiatric and psychological factors also render persons more vulnerable, some of which are the key comorbidities of substance use disorders. Personality factors make people more risk seeking, more likely to experiment with behaviors, and more sensitive to rewards, therefore more sensitive to the reinforcing properties of drugs and less sensitive to the consequences of drug use. Others are consequence and risk avoidant, and are relatively protected from addiction. Depression 'turns off' the reward system so that ordinary rewards of life are less reinforcing, and people become more sensitive to the rewarding effects of drugs. Life experiences that expose people to drugs and social acceptance of drug use also increase the risk of addiction. Finally, biology is involved in several ways. In the case of alcoholism, genetic makeup affects the degree to which alcohol is rewarding. Some patients tell you that their first drink was so rewarding they began a lifetime of heavy drinking immediately. Others say they never really liked drinking all that much, and therefore are surprised as they become more and more dependent on alcohol to control the emotional discomforts of their lives. Cocaine-related reward is less affected by genetics, and patients with exposure to cocaine describe intense pleasure. However, cocaine dependence is more affected by the genetics of risk taking and reward sensitivity that shape personality [9]. Finally, medical conditions such as chronic pain, a variety of disease states and surgical procedures may result in exposure to addictive drugs and may amplify their reinforcing effects. Such patients may develop iatrogenic addiction, and then persistent drug use problems. All of these factors enhance or diminish the risk of the cycle getting out of control.

Finally, choice involves the free will of the individual to initiate and continue using the drug (although Skinner did not believe in free will). Choice becomes narrower as addiction progresses by way of stronger drive and conditioned learning, but it is only through the individual's choice that treatment and change can begin.

A Behavioral Approach to the Treatment of Chronic Pain

Nearly all the patients referred to the pain treatment program at the Johns Hopkins Hospital exhibit elements of both conditioned pain behaviors and addictive behaviors. The treatment of these patients has usually been very unsuccessful because of both complex pain pathology and complex psychiatric comorbidity. All patients need a careful expert evaluation of their medical problem. The diagnostic formulation should look at the whole person in the context of his or her life, as well as at the burdens of their pathologies.

Ideally, chronic pain should be cured or relieved completely. Unfortunately, chronic pain usually is the result of a multifactorial dysregulation of the many systems involved in sensing and reacting to pain. There is crosstalk between the sensory and autonomic apparatus at every level of pain transmission. Sensory elements of pain can be altered at the nociceptor apparatus and at every synapse all the way to the thalamus and cortex. The emotional elements of pain are likewise complex and open to modification. Pain amplification syndromes are complex and involve almost continuous adaptation. Even the most straightforward models of pain continue to surprise us with their complexity. While we tend to categorize pain as neuropathic, central, sympathetically maintained and others, these conditions have overlap in most patients who are refractory to treatment. After a complete workup for treatable underlying pathologies responsible for the pain, we use a behaviorally based interdisciplinary approach to pain.

This process begins with the identification of physical and psychiatric conditions that contribute to the problem. Key comorbidities include depression, personality disorder, and family and social factors that all play a role in the disabling chronic pain disorder. Intoxication with benzodiazepines and opiates (often others), opiate-mediated hyperalgesia, deconditioning, chronic constipation, poor nutrition (or even cachexia), vitamin deficiency, endocrine dysregulation including hypotestosteronemia, hypothyroidism and steroid dependence are commonly seen comorbidities. These all must be described to the patient (usually repeatedly as they are often intoxicated at first) and incorporated into the treatment plan.

The rehabilitation part of our treatment program uses group therapy, a structured milieu, active physical therapy and reconditioning, and cognitive behavioral therapy. We engage any treatment modality beneficial to function (local blocks, transcutaneous electrical nerve stimulation units, spinal cord stimulators, biofeedback, structured relaxation, massage when available and acupuncture when available), provided these contribute to improved engagement in rehabilitation. We treat pain with a variety of pharmacological interventions, but do not use any reinforcing medications (e.g. benzodiazepines, barbiturates, muscle relaxants, opioids). We employ tricyclic antidepressants, serotonin-norepinephrine reuptake inhibitor antidepressants, anticonvulsants, nonsteroidal anti-inflammatory drugs, topical lidocaine, capsaicin, salicylate topicals and numerous other medications based on type of pain and other factors.

The behavioral elements of treatment are similar to those laid out by William Fordyce in the 1970s. First, behaviors are selected that need to be changed, and reinforcers that will be salient to the patient are determined. Often family members must change behaviors that act as reinforcers of the illness behaviors the patient exhibits.

1 Analyze behavior and reinforcers
2 Select reinforcers
3 Develop goals
4 Extinguish pain behaviors
5 Reinforce healthy behaviors
6 Add reinforcers and expand healthy behaviors

While the reason for abnormal gaits, odd postures, distorted eating behaviors and odd bowel habits may be physiological, we use physical therapy, occupational therapy and rehabilitation directed at correcting these to the degree physiologically possible. Pain medications such as nonsteroidal anti-inflammatory drugs and acetaminophen are nonreinforcing, but all reinforcing medications are given by schedule rather than as needed. The exception is for withdrawal symptoms that may compromise health, which is when we adjust the schedule to avoid additional PRN medications as much as possible. We use nonreinforcing medications to ameliorate withdrawal generously, but some behaviorists feel that no PRN medications should be used as the act of coping with noxious sensations using medication is being reinforced.

A variety of reinforcers have been particularly useful to us in our work, including all four of the types described in the figure on operant conditioning (fig. 1). Patients are differentially responsive to reinforcement, some being more consequence avoidant and others more reward seeking. Each patient needs ongoing monitoring of results and ongoing adjustment of the treatment plan. In table 4, we have included some interventions we find useful. We discuss these with the patient and tend to be very transparent about our behavioral techniques. Patients may play an active role in selecting reinforcers as they get better. There are relatively few punishments because our patients tend to be reward responsive rather than punishment responsive. We require all patients to attend groups, therapy sessions and ward activities. We gradually impose more behavioral incentives if patients do not cooperate. We are extremely sympathetic with the discomforts patients must tolerate, but do not excuse them from treatment activities based on feelings. We focus on behaviors rather than feelings and progress rather than limitations.

Table 4. Operant conditioning paradigm (as shown in table 1) applied to treatment of patients with chronic pain

		Stimulus quality	
		positive	negative
Stimulus when behavior occurs	deliver	*Positive reinforcement* privileges; attention and praise; promotion to better settings; special food; access to specialists; access to tests and resources; letters to lawyers; legitimacy (behavior increases)	*Punishment* restriction; informing outsiders of lack of cooperation; discharge; (behavior decreases)
	withdraw	*Extinction* increasing rate of taper; decreasing time of therapy; refusal to order tests and consults; refusal to provide resources; discharge; ignoring the behavior and the patient (behavior decreases)	*Negative reinforcement* relief from distress; relief from outside criticism; removal of restriction; removal of pressure to get medication; relief from responsibilities (behavior increases)

Addiction can be defined as the process of the cycle gradually getting out of control and losing the usual controls. It is obvious that most people who are exposed to addictive substances do not become addicted. To treat addiction requires that the clinician address not only the host (patient) factors that make the person vulnerable (depression, personality issues, life circumstances), but also the behavioral loop that is now out of control and driving the behavior independently of the initiating factors. As above, we approach addictive behaviors using a behavioral model. We often require patients with strong elements of addictive behavior to attend 12-step-based groups as these groups also focus on behaviors to be accomplished (steps) rather than feelings to be achieved.

Conclusions

Pain is a complex symptom involving both sensory and emotional experiences. Chronic pain may change over time, and has elements of conditioned behavior in many cases. Opiate treatment of chronic pain is frequently problematic and may result in addictive behaviors, which then exacerbate the conditioning elements of the pain and its disability. A comprehensive approach to rehabilitation of patients disordered by chronic pain includes a strong element of behaviorist methodology. Often function can be restored with a comprehensive program including pain treatment and behavioral change. The reinforcing role of some aspects of the current culture contribute to the disorder of vulnerable patients and play a role in the development of addictive behaviors.

References

1 Fordyce WE, Fowler RS, DeLateur B: An application of behavior modification technique to a problem of chronic pain. Behav Res Ther 1968;6:105–107.
2 Pilowsky I: Abnormal illness behaviour. Br J Med Psychol 1969;42:347–351.
3 Roscoe JA, Morrow GR, Aapro MS, Molassiotis A, Olver I: Anticipatory nausea and vomiting. Support Care Cancer 2010, E-pub ahead of print.
4 Poulos CX, Hinson RE, Siegel S: The role of Pavlovian processes in drug tolerance and dependence: implications for treatment. Addict Behav 1981;6:205–211.
5 Skinner BF: The operant side of behavior therapy. J Behav Ther Exp Psychiatry 1988;19:171–179.
6 Turk DC, Okifuji A: What factors affect physicians' decisions to prescribe opioids for chronic noncancer pain patients? Clin J Pain 1997;13:330–336.
7 Bekhit MH: Opioid-induced hyperalgesia and tolerance. Am J Ther 2010;17:498–510.
8 McHugh PR, Slavney PR: The Perspectives of Psychiatry, ed 2. Baltimore, JHU, 1998.
9 Schuckit MA: An overview of genetic influences in alcoholism. J Subst Abuse Treat 2009;36:S5–S14.

Glenn J. Treisman, MD, PhD
Department of Psychiatry and Behavioral Sciences
Meyer 110, The Johns Hopkins Hospital, 600 North Wolfe Street
Baltimore, MD 21287 (USA)
Tel. +1 410 955 6328, E-Mail glenn@jhmi.edu

Clark MR, Treisman GJ (eds): Chronic Pain and Addiction.
Adv Psychosom Med. Basel, Karger, 2011, vol 30, pp 22–60

Addiction and Brain Reward and Antireward Pathways

Eliot L. Gardner

Neuropsychopharmacology Section, Intramural Research Program, National Institute on Drug Abuse,
National Institutes of Health, Baltimore, Md., USA

Abstract

Addictive drugs have in common that they are voluntarily self-administered by laboratory animals (usually avidly), and that they enhance the functioning of the reward circuitry of the brain (producing the 'high' that the drug user seeks). The core reward circuitry consists of an 'in-series' circuit linking the ventral tegmental area, nucleus accumbens and ventral pallidum via the medial forebrain bundle. Although originally believed to simply encode the set point of hedonic tone, these circuits are now believed to be functionally far more complex, also encoding attention, expectancy of reward, disconfirmation of reward expectancy, and incentive motivation. 'Hedonic dysregulation' within these circuits may lead to addiction. The 'second-stage' dopaminergic component in this reward circuitry is the crucial addictive-drug-sensitive component. All addictive drugs have in common that they enhance (directly or indirectly or even transsynaptically) dopaminergic reward synaptic function in the nucleus accumbens. Drug self-administration is regulated by nucleus accumbens dopamine levels, and is done to keep nucleus accumbens dopamine within a specific elevated range (to maintain a desired hedonic level). For some classes of addictive drugs (e.g. opiates), tolerance to the euphoric effects develops with chronic use. Postuse dysphoria then comes to dominate reward circuit hedonic tone, and addicts no longer use drugs to get high, but simply to get back to normal ('get straight'). The brain circuits mediating the pleasurable effects of addictive drugs are anatomically, neurophysiologically and neurochemically different from those mediating physical dependence, and from those mediating craving and relapse. There are important genetic variations in vulnerability to drug addiction, yet environmental factors such as stress and social defeat also alter brain-reward mechanisms in such a manner as to impart vulnerability to addiction. In short, the 'bio-psycho-social' model of etiology holds very well for addiction. Addiction appears to correlate with a hypodopaminergic dysfunctional state within the reward circuitry of the brain. Neuroimaging studies in humans add credence to this hypothesis. Credible evidence also implicates serotonergic, opioid, endocannabinoid, GABAergic and glutamatergic mechanisms in addiction. Critically, drug addiction progresses from occasional recreational use to impulsive use to habitual compulsive use. This correlates with a progression from reward-driven to habit-driven drug-seeking behavior. This behavioral progression correlates with a neuroanatomical progression from ventral striatal (nucleus accumbens) to dorsal striatal control over drug-seeking behavior. The three classical sets of craving and relapse triggers are (a) reexposure to addictive drugs, (b) stress, and (c) reexposure to environmental cues (people, places, things) previously associated with drug-taking behavior. Drug-triggered relapse involves the nucleus accumbens and the neurotransmitter dopamine. Stress-triggered relapse involves (a) the central nucleus of the amygdala, the bed nucleus of the stria terminalis, and the neurotransmitter corticotrophin-releasing factor, and (b) the lateral tegmental noradrenergic nuclei of the brain stem and the neurotransmitter norepinephrine. Cue-triggered relapse involves the basolateral nucleus of the amygdala, the hippocampus and the neurotransmitter glutamate. Knowledge of the neuroanatomy, neurophysiology, neurochemistry and neuropharmacology of addictive drug action in the brain is currently producing a variety of strategies for pharmacotherapeutic treatment of drug addiction, some of which appear promising.

Addiction – An Age-Old Medical and Societal Problem

The abusive use of addictive drugs is a medical and societal problem as old as recorded human history. One particularly ancient reference to it may be found in the Hebrew/Christian Bible, where in Genesis, chapter 9, verses 20–23, the Semite Patriarch Noah is described as becoming drunken, disheveled, naked and filthy from overindulgence in wine. Similarly ancient references to drug abuse may be found in the oral and written traditions of virtually all ethnic and cultural groups on the planet.

One of the most striking features of drug addiction is how few chemicals are subject to abuse. If one takes all congeners of all known chemicals, approximately 30,000,000 chemical substances are known [1]. Yet, only approximately 100 (including nicotine, ethanol, psychostimulants, opiates, barbiturates, benzodiazepines and cannabinoids) are addictive. In truth, 100 is a stunningly small subset of 30,000,000. It poses the question: what makes those 100 chemicals addictive, while the remaining 30,000,000 chemicals lack this property? After all, upon cursory examination, there seem few pharmacological similarities among addictive drugs. Some – including barbiturates, ethanol, opiates and benzodiazepines – are sedatives, while others – including nicotine, cocaine and the amphetamines – are stimulants. Some – including opiates and cannabinoids – are antinociceptive, while others (in the proper laboratory or clinical situations) are pronociceptive. Some – such as ethanol and opiates – produce striking degrees of physical dependence, while others – such as cocaine – produce little if any physical dependence. However, a few commonalities are both apparent and instructive. All addictive drugs are subjectively rewarding, reinforcing and pleasurable [1]. Laboratory animals volitionally self-administer them [2], just as humans do. Furthermore, the rank order of appetitiveness in animals parallels the rank order of appetitiveness in humans [2, 3]. Most tellingly, perhaps, all addictive drugs (with the exception of the LSD-like and mescaline-like hallucinogens) activate the reward circuitry of the brain [1, 4, 5], thereby producing the subjective 'high' that the drug abuser seeks. Furthermore, the degree of such activation of the brain's reward circuitry correlates well with the degree of subjective high.

The Brain's Reward Circuitry

The brain's reward circuitry was first discovered by Olds and Milner [6] at McGill University in the early 1950s. They found that animals would repeatedly return to an area of the laboratory in which they had received mild electrical stimulation of subcortical structures anatomically associated with the medial forebrain bundle. Subsequently, they found that animals would avidly perform tasks (e.g. depressing wall-mounted levers in their test chambers) in order to receive such brain stimulation. In the aftermath of this discovery of the phenomenon of brain stimulation reward, Olds and Olds [7–10] carried out extensive mapping studies of the rodent brain, confirming that a large majority of the brain sites supporting brain stimulation reward are associated with the nuclei of origin, tracts and terminal loci of the medial forebrain bundle. Other researchers [11] studied electrical brain stimulation reward in nonhuman primates and confirmed that the anatomic brain substrates in primates were homologous to those in rodents. Using sophisticated electrophysiological techniques, Gallistel et al. [12] determined that the primary neural substrate supporting electrical brain stimulation reward is the moderately fast-conducting, myelinated descending neural fiber system of the medial forebrain bundle. This system originates in the anterior bed nuclei of the medial forebrain bundle (an array of deep subcortical limbic loci anterior to the hypothalamus and preoptic area), descends to the ventral tegmental area of the midbrain via the medial forebrain bundle, and then ascends via the medial forebrain bundle to a select group of forebrain limbic loci including the nucleus accumbens, olfactory tubercle and frontal cortex. Wise and Bozarth [13] were the first to realize that this assortment of brain loci and tracts constituted a neural circuit containing three synaptically connected, in-series neuronal elements: a descending link running from the anterior bed nuclei of the medial forebrain bundle to the ventral tegmental area, an ascending link running from the ventral tegmental area to the nucleus accumbens, and a further ascending link running from the nucleus accumbens to the ventral pallidum. The first link is the descending myelinated fiber tract first identified by Gallistel et al. [12], of unknown neurotransmitter type, although very recent evidence raises, by inference, the possibility that glutamate in the ventral tegmental area might play a role [14]. The second link is the ascending fiber tract from the ventral tegmental area to the nucleus accumbens, with dopamine as its neurotransmitter (see below). The third link is the projection from the nucleus accumbens to the ventral pallidum, using γ-aminobutyric acid (GABA), substance P and enkephalin as conjoint neurotransmitters [15–22]. This three-neuron, in-series circuit receives synaptic inputs from, and is functionally modulated by, a wide variety of other neural circuits including cholinergic, endorphinergic, serotonergic, GABAergic, glutamatergic, enkephalinergic, dynorphinergic and substance P-containing neural elements [1].

Addictive drugs of different classes act on this three-neuron, in-series brain reward neural circuit at different points to activate the circuit and produce the drug-induced high. Barbiturates, benzodiazepines, cannabinoids, ethanol, nicotine and opiates act on synapses associated with the ventral tegmental area. Amphetamines, cannabinoids, cocaine, opiates and dissociative anesthetics such as ketamine and phencyclidine act on synapses associated with the nucleus accumbens [1–3, 5].

Importantly, this brain reward circuitry (fig. 1) evolved over eons of evolution to subserve biologically essential normal rewarding behaviors such as feeding, drinking, sexual behavior, maternal and paternal behaviors, and social interactions. The reinforcement engendered by such normal reward is believed to underlie the consolidation of biologically essential memories (e.g. food and water location within an animal's foraging or hunting range) [23]. After all, it is teleological thinking at its most tendentious and intellectually vacuous to imagine that these circuits emerged through hundreds of millions of years of vertebrate and mammalian evolution simply so that 21st-century humans can imbibe, inhale or inject themselves with addictive drugs [1]. From an appreciation of the natural and biologically essential nature of the functioning of these reward circuits comes the notion that addictive drugs 'hijack' the brain's reward circuits, activating them more strongly than natural rewards, and diverting the drug addict's life to pursuit of drug-induced pleasure at the expense of 'getting off' on life's normal pleasures and rewards [24, 25].

The Intense Nature of Brain Stimulation Reward

Electrical brain stimulation reward is remarkable for the intensity of the reward and reinforcement produced [1]. When the stimulating electrode is properly on target within the ventral tegmental area, medial forebrain bundle or nucleus accumbens, laboratory animals will volitionally self-stimulate those areas at maximal rates. They will, tellingly, ignore readily available food, water, toys and sexually receptive animals of the opposite sex in order to self-deliver the brain stimulation reward. They will also volitionally accept aversive and painful consequences in order to self-deliver the brain stimulation reward. In awake humans, such electrical stimulation can evoke intense subjective feelings of pleasure [26–31], in some instances similar to descriptions of intense medieval religious ecstasies [Ward A.A. Jr., pers. commun., 1967]. As the most addictive drugs (e.g. cocaine, methamphetamine) evoke comparable levels of subjective reward, it is easy to understand their intensely addictive nature.

Using Electrical Brain Stimulation Reward to Assess the Degree of Reward Evoked by Addictive Drugs

In the half-century since the initial discovery of the brain stimulation reward phenomenon, a number of techniques have been developed to quantify the degree of reward enhancement produced by addictive drugs. Using simple rate-based

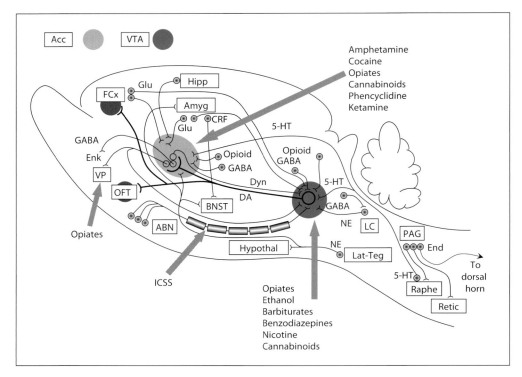

Fig. 1. Diagram of the brain reward circuitry of the mammalian (laboratory rat) brain, with sites at which various addictive drugs act to enhance brain reward mechanisms and thus to produce drug-seeking behavior, drug-taking behavior, drug craving and relapse to drug-seeking behavior. ABN = Anterior bed nuclei of the medial forebrain bundle; Acc = nucleus accumbens; Amyg = amygdala; BNST = bed nucleus of the stria terminalis; CRF = corticotrophin-releasing factor; DA = subcomponent of the ascending mesocorticolimbic dopaminergic system that appears to be preferentially activated by addictive drugs; Dyn = dynorphinergic neuronal fiber bundle outflow from the nucleus accumbens; Enk = enkephalinergic neuronal fiber bundle outflow from the nucleus accumbens; FCx = frontal cortex; GABA = GABAergic inhibitory fiber systems synapsing in the ventral tegmental area, in the nucleus accumbens and into the vicinity of the locus ceruleus, as well as the GABAergic neuronal fiber bundle outflow from the nucleus accumbens; Glu = glutamatergic neural systems originating in the frontal cortex and synapsing in both the ventral tegmental area and the nucleus accumbens; 5-HT = serotonergic (5-hydroxytryptamine) fibers, which originate in the anterior raphe nuclei and project to both the cell body region (ventral tegmental area) and terminal projection field (nucleus accumbens) of the DA reward neurons; ICSS = descending, myelinated, moderately fast-conducting component of the brain reward circuitry that is preferentially activated by electrical intracranial self-stimulation (electrical brain stimulation reward); LC = locus ceruleus; NE = noradrenergic fibers, which originate in the locus ceruleus and synapse into the general vicinity of the ventral mesencephalic neuronal cell fields of the ventral tegmental area; Opioid = endogenous opioid peptide neural systems synapsing into both the ventral tegmental DA cell fields and the nucleus accumbens DA terminal projection loci; PAG = periaqueductal gray matter; Raphe = brainstem serotonergic raphe nuclei; VP = ventral pallidum; VTA = ventral tegmental area. After Gardner [1].

measures (e.g. how rapidly a test animal lever-presses or nose-pokes to receive brain stimulation reward) is unsatisfactory as many addictive drugs have either motor-stimulating or -depressant properties. Rate-independent test paradigms are essential. One of the earliest rate-independent paradigms was the 2-lever titrating threshold paradigm [32]. In this paradigm, the test animal depresses a wall-mounted primary lever in its test chamber to receive the brain stimulation, which decreases by a preset amount (either in amperes or hertz) with each successive stimulation. At some point, the stimulation decreases to a level insufficient to activate the neurons at the tip of the implanted electrode in the brain, the consequence of which is that the animal ceases to experience the subjective reward or pleasure evoked by the stimulation. At this point, the animal presses a wall-mounted secondary lever, which delivers no brain stimulation, but merely resets the brain stimulator back to its original intensity. By assessing the mean reset level, one obtains a rate-independent (and, thus, motor impairment- or motor stimulation-free) measure of brain reward function. As monkeys (and even some laboratory rats) are clever enough to adopt an alternating lever-pressing pattern of behavior to keep the brain stimulation intensity at a maximum, a variant of the technique was developed, in which the resetting of stimulation intensity is controlled by withholding of response on the primary lever [33]. Since animals volitionally self-stimulate at even marginally rewarding levels of stimulation, this technique yields rate-independent threshold measures of brain reward intensity that appear to track the rewarding-enhancing properties of addictive drugs with accuracy and consistency.

Another rate-independent brain stimulation reward measuring technique commonly used in recent decades is the rate-frequency (or, alternatively, rate-amperage) curve-shift method [34, 35]. In this paradigm, the test animal has only a single manipulandum (e.g. lever, nose-poke detector) in its test chamber, the activation of which delivers the rewarding brain stimulation (usually with a duration of 250 ms). A test session consists of a successive series of short 'bins' of opportunity to self-stimulate (e.g. 20 s), each bin being at a lower intensity of stimulation. As the hertz (or amperage level) decreases, the stimulation decreases to a level insufficient to activate the neurons at the tip of the implanted electrode in the brain, and the animal ceases to experience the subjective reward, leading to a fairly abrupt cessation of responding. By plotting stimulation frequency (or amperage) against rate of responding, one obtains a rate-independent measure of brain reward function. A typical rate-frequency or rate-amperage plot is sigmoidal in shape and can be conceptualized in the same way as a dose-response curve in classical pharmacology. As in classical pharmacology, a left-shift constitutes an enhancement of efficacy (in this case, an intensification of brain reward) and a right-shift constitutes a diminution of efficacy (an inhibition of brain reward).

Using the rate-frequency curve-shift brain stimulation reward paradigm, much work has been devoted to assessing the brain reward-enhancing properties of addictive drugs. With the exception of nicotine (which is inexplicably powerful at

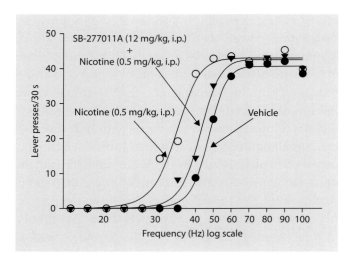

Fig. 2. Left-shift with addictive drug, countered by selective D$_3$ receptor antagonist.

enhancing electrical brain reward functions), the degree of enhancement of brain reward by addictive drugs nicely parallels the degree of subjective high experienced by human users of such drugs [1]. The action of nicotine on brain reward is intriguing. According to most cigarette smokers, nicotine does not produce a powerful subjective high. Yet, nicotine is the most addictive chemical known [36]. Is it possible that the action of nicotine in the electrical brain stimulation reward paradigm is more congruent with its addictive potency than with its potency on the subjective experience of high? That seems counterintuitive, yet it would appear that such a possibility must be entertained.

These methods can also be used to assess the degree to which potential antiaddiction pharmacotherapeutic medications attenuate addictive drug-enhanced brain reward, and thus, by inference, the degree to which such putatively therapeutic agents might attenuate addictive drug-induced highs in human drug abusers (fig. 2) [37–41]. These methods can also be used to study the brain mechanisms underlying the 'low dose-good trip/high dose-bad trip' subjective phenomenon often reported by drug addicts. Similar to human reports, animals also appear to experience enhancement of brain reward at low-to-moderate doses of addictive drugs, while experiencing inhibition of reward at high doses of the same drugs [42, 43].

Activation of Brain Reward Substrates by Direct Intracerebral Microinjection of Addictive Drugs

Just as systemic injections of addictive drugs enhance brain reward substrates, so too does intracerebral microinjection. Compellingly, the brain sites that support intracerebral microinjections of addictive drugs are, by and large, the same brain sites that support electrical brain stimulation reward [1, 2, 5, 13]. Thus, it may be inferred that common neural substrates underlie reward enhancement induced by addictive drugs, however administered. This is an important component of the conception that addictive drugs derive their addictive action from enhancement of brain reward mechanisms.

Another technique for measuring the rewarding properties of addictive drugs is that of conditioned place preference/aversion [44–46]. In the most simple variant of this animal model, a two-compartment test chamber is used, each compartment having distinctly different environmental cues (e.g. one compartment with striped walls, a smooth floor and lemon odor, the other compartment with plain walls, a rough floor and pine scent). Between the two compartments is a vertical sliding door which, when in place, prevents movement from one compartment to the other. The animal is initially placed in the chamber with the door absent, thus allowing free passage back and forth between both compartments. The environmental cues have previously been adjusted so that on initial exposure to the test chamber, animals show no inherent preference for one compartment over the other. On the next day, the door is inserted, blocking passage between the compartments. The animal is administered a drug, enough time is allowed to elapse so that the peak drug effect is reached, and the animal is placed into one cue-distinct compartment for a modest period of time (e.g. 15 min). On the next test day, the animal is administered vehicle and placed into the other cue-distinct compartment for the same length of time. On successive days, animals alternate between the drug-paired and vehicle-paired compartments. This 'training' goes on for approximately 10 days (i.e. 5 days being given the drug and placed in the drug-paired, cue-distinct compartment, and 5 days being given vehicle and placed in the vehicle-paired, cue-distinct compartment). The next day is the 'test' day, on which the door is once again removed, allowing free passage between compartments, and the test animal is not administered anything. If the animal volitionally spends a disproportionate amount of time in the formerly drug-paired compartment, it is inferred that the animal is displaying drug-seeking behavior, and it is further inferred that the drug experience must have been rewarding. If the animal volitionally spends a disproportionate amount of time in the formerly vehicle-paired compartment, it is inferred that the animal is displaying drug-avoidance behavior, and it is further inferred that the drug experience must have been aversive. Compellingly, the only drugs that consistently produce place preference rather than place neutrality or place aversion are addictive drugs [46]. Equally compellingly, place preference is evoked by intracerebral microinjections of addictive drugs by and large into the same brain sites that support electrical brain stimulation reward and support volitional intracerebral self-microinjection of addictive drugs [5]. This is yet another important component of the conception that addictive drugs derive their addictive action from enhancement of brain reward mechanisms.

The Crucial Reward Neurotransmitter in the Brain Is Dopamine

The crucial brain reward neurotransmitter activated by addictive drugs is dopamine, specifically in the 'second-stage' ventral tegmental area to nucleus accumbens link in the brain's reward circuitry. This has been learned over many decades of research, and is based upon many congruent findings.

First, virtually all addictive drugs are functional dopamine agonists – some direct, some indirect, some even transsynaptic [1, 4, 5]. In fact, with the exception of the LSD- and mescaline-like hallucinogens, functional dopamine agonism is the single pharmacological property that all addictive drugs share. Second, intracerebral micro-injections of dopamine agonists produce conditioned place preference (see discussion above) and support volitional intracerebral self-administration [5]. Third, dopamine antagonists are negative reinforcers in animals (animals will work to avoid or escape their administration) and produce subjectively aversive effects in humans [1, 3]. Fourth, when dopamine antagonists are administered to animals volitionally self-administering addictive drugs, a compensatory increase in addictive drug intake occurs (to compensate for the decreased rewarding potency of the addictive drug), followed by extinction and cessation of the self-administration behavior (when the dopamine antagonism reaches a sufficient intensity so as to totally block the rewarding properties of the self-administered addictive drug) [3, 47]. Fifth, measures of real-time synaptic neurochemistry in the nucleus accumbens of test animals volitionally engaged in intravenous self-administration of addictive drugs (the real-time neurochemical sampling being achieved by in vivo brain microdialysis [48]) show that: (a) following the first volitional self-administration of the test session, extracellular dopamine overflow in the nucleus accumbens displays a tonic increase of approximately 200%; (b) thereafter, extracellular dopamine levels in the nucleus accumbens fluctuate phasically between approximately 200 and 100% over baseline, and (c) the low point of each phasic dip in extracellular nucleus accumbens dopamine accurately predicts the next volitional intake of addictive drug by the test animal (fig. 3) [49–51].

Brain Antireward Systems and Addiction – Proponent and Opponent Brain Reward Processes

Drawing on Solomon's hypothesis about the existence of proponent and opponent motivational processes [52–54], Koob et al. [55–57] have proposed that there are similar proponent and opponent processes at work in the brain substrates of reward [1]. The proponent brain reward processes are hypothesized to produce enhancement of brain reward, and to show development of tolerance over time. The opponent brain reward processes are hypothesized to produce inhibition of brain reward, and to show progressive enhancement of strength over time. The proponent (proreward) and opponent (antireward) processes are hypothesized

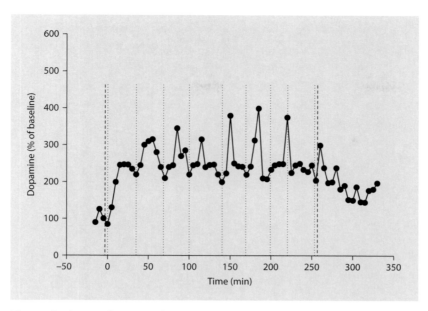

Fig. 3. Real-time dopamine brain microdialysis during intravenous opiate self-administration. Courtesy of Dr. Roy A. Wise.

to occur simultaneously and to functionally oppose each other in a mutually inhibitory fashion. Using electrical brain stimulation reward in laboratory rodents, Gardner and Lowinson [42] and Nazzaro et al. [58] reported finding proreward and antireward processes that correspond remarkably well to Koob's hypothesized proponent and opponent brain reward mechanisms. Gardner and Lowinson [42] and Broderick et al. [59, 60] reported finding similar proreward and antireward processes measured neurochemically by in vivo brain electrochemistry (in vivo voltammetry) in laboratory rodents.

As can be readily seen from an inspection of figure 4, these proreward and antireward mechanisms have important implications for understanding the nature of the overall shift in reward level or hedonic tone produced by addictive drugs. If the reward-enhancing effect shown in figure 4a is combined with the reward-inhibiting effect shown in figure 4b, it appears that administration of an opiate (in this case morphine) initially produces a strong enhancement of brain reward (the high) that is countered by only a weak simultaneous antireward process. The net effect on brain reward or subjective hedonic tone is significant reward enhancement (high). However, with repeated opiate administration, the proreward mechanism depicted in figure 4a progressively diminishes, while the antireward mechanism depicted in figure 4b grows progressively stronger. Thus, with repeated opiate administration, the overall net effect on hedonic tone becomes more and more inhibitory since the opponent processes grow stronger and are opposed by progressively weaker

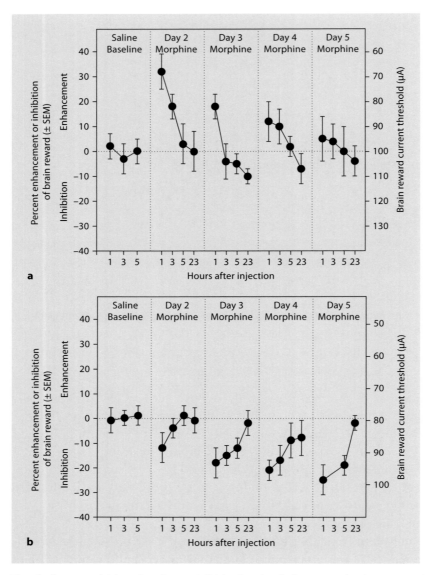

Fig. 4. Proreward (**a**) and antireward (**b**) brain stimulation reward substrates activated by opiate administration. From Nazzaro et al. [58].

proponent processes. Gardner [1] and Gardner and David [4] proposed that this may constitute at least a partial mechanistic explanation for the frequent report by human heroin addicts that – after having lived with the disease of opiate addiction for some time – they no longer self-administer heroin to get high, but rather to simply get straight (i.e. to push their diminished subjective hedonic tone back towards normality).

Brain Antireward Systems and Addiction – Brain Reward Processes during Withdrawal

As noted above, brain reward is enhanced by acute administration of addictive drugs. Conversely, in withdrawal, brain reward is inhibited, sometimes profoundly. This was first reported by Kokkinidis and McCarter [61] in 1990 – using the electrical brain stimulation reward paradigm in laboratory rodents – and has been amply confirmed since [62–65]. These robust inhibitory effects on brain reward would appear to constitute the mechanistic neural substrate of the inhibition of hedonic tone experienced by drug addicts during withdrawal. It should be well noted that this hedonic withdrawal state is unrelated to the physical withdrawal state experienced concomitantly by addicts experiencing acute withdrawal (e.g. cramps, diarrhea and physical pain during opiate withdrawal).

Brain Antireward Systems and Addiction – 'Reward Deficiency' as a Driving Force in Addiction

In 1996, Blum et al. [66, 67] proposed that many aspects of addiction are driven by a chronic basal deficiency in brain reward which mechanistically underlies a chronic basal deficiency in subjective hedonic tone. This hypothesis has been amplified and expanded, both by its original proponents and by others [68–71]. The fundamental notion is a simple one: that drug addicts are either born with or acquire a deficiency state in the dopaminergic brain substrates of reward and positive hedonic tone, and turn to addictive drug use to remedy this chronic reward deficiency. Thus, the reward deficiency hypothesis seeks to explain drug addiction as a type of self-medication, ultimately damaging and self-destructive though it may be. The brain substrate of this reward deficiency syndrome may be mechanistically referable to more than a single deficiency in the functioning of the brain's dopaminergic reward circuitry. Comings and Blum [70] and Blum et al. [72] have hypothesized that it is referable to a deficiency of dopaminergic D_2 receptors in the brain's reward circuitry, a view congruent with reports – including neuroimaging of the brain – by Volkow et al. [73–76], Nader and colleagues [77], and Everitt and colleagues [78], among others. Staley and Mash [79], Mash [80], Gardner and colleagues [46, 81–83], Heidbreder et al. [84, 85] and others have hypothesized that it may be referable to an aberration in dopaminergic D_3 receptors in the brain's reward circuitry.

Nestler and Kosten and colleagues [86, 87] have hypothesized that it may be referable to a deficiency in presynaptic dopamine levels in the reward-crucial nucleus accumbens. They initially arrived at this hypothesis from studying laboratory rodents made vulnerable to drug addiction (i.e. exhibiting a high preference for addictive drugs and high drug-seeking behavior) by two quite different means, one genetic and one experiential. By selective breeding, it is possible to genetically select for the behavioral phenotype of high addictive drug preference and high addictive drug-seeking behavior [88–93]. Conversely, it is equally possible to genetically select for the behavioral phenotype of addictive drug avoidance and low addictive drug-seeking behavior. While some of these strains have been deliberately bred, it has also been recognized that some rodent strains have acquired these converse behavioral phenotypes during natural evolution. In this regard, the Lewis and Fischer 344 rat strains are notable. Lewis rats are naturally highly addictive-drug-preferring and drug-seeking. Fischer 344 rats are naturally highly addictive-drug-avoidant. It is also possible to confer the behavioral phenotype of high addictive drug preference and high addictive drug-seeking behavior by experiential means, i.e. by exposing animals to repeated administration of addictive drugs. Nestler and Kosten and colleagues [86, 87] studied the dopaminergic brain reward circuits of laboratory rats made vulnerable (or resistant) to addictive drugs by both genetic and experiential means. They found that in animals displaying the behavioral phenotype of high addictive drug acceptance and high addictive drug seeking – whether this behavioral phenotype was imparted genetically or experientially – there exists a pathological atrophy of the neurofilamentous transport system for the dopamine-synthesizing enzyme tyrosine hydroxylase in the dopamine axons of the second-stage medial forebrain bundle neurons of the brain's reward circuitry. Congruently, they found a pathological deficiency in tyrosine hydroxylase in the dopaminergic axon terminals of the nucleus accumbens, a pathological deficiency of extracellular dopamine in the nucleus accumbens, and concomitant pathological aberrations in postreceptor transduction mechanisms (e.g. adenylate cyclase, cyclic AMP, protein kinase A) in the next-following postsynaptic neurons, all in comparison to control animals not displaying the addictive drug-accepting and drug-seeking behavioral phenotype.

As a result of such findings, Gardner [1] hypothesized that some drug addicts may 'have a defect in their ability to capture reward and pleasure from everyday experience', and noted that this has been hypothesized by astute clinicians for more than 45 years [94, 95]. Gardner [1] has further noted that 'if this be so, then our goals are really two-fold: first, to rescue addicts from the clutches of their addictions, and second, to restore their reward systems to a level of functionality that will enable them to "get off" on the real world'.

The Functional Roles of the Crucial Nucleus Accumbens Reward Neurons

Based upon an extensive review of the literature regarding brain reward mechanisms, Wise [96] suggested more than 30 years ago that 'the dopamine junction [in the nucleus accumbens] represents a synaptic way station for messages signaling the rewarding impact of a variety of normally powerful rewarding events. It seems likely that this synapse lies at a critical junction between the branches of the sensory pathways which carry signals of the intensity, duration, and quality of the stimulus, and the motivational pathways where these sensory inputs are translated into the hedonic messages we experience as pleasure, euphoria, or "yumminess'" [96]. While this remains an appropriate description of the role of the reward circuitry in encoding hedonic tone, an extraordinary amount of electrophysiological, neurochemical and behavioral neuroscience research over the last 20 years has made it apparent that the crucial nucleus accumbens reward neurons do more than encode receipt of reward, although encoding receipt of reward is certainly one of their functions [97]. They also appear (1) to encode expectancy of reward [98, 99], amount of reward [98], delay of reward [100], reward delay discounting [101] and errors in reward prediction [102]; (2) to regulate motivation for drug-seeking behavior [103], and (3) to contribute to the synaptic neuroplasticity that underlies the acquisition of addictive behavior patterns [104].

Genetic and Experiential Contributions to the Disease of Addiction

As noted above, it is relatively easy to selectively breed laboratory animals for the behavioral phenotype of drug-seeking behavior (the behavioral phenotype breeds true after about 15 generations in laboratory rodents). At the human level, family, adoption and twin studies have consistently demonstrated a substantial genetic influence in the development of drug addiction, with inherited risk estimates ranging between 40 and 60% [105, 106]. The exact role of individual genes in this complex disease is not yet fully characterized, but the contribution of genetics to addiction is generally thought to be polygenic, with multiple low-impact genes combining to create the genetic vulnerability [107]. Just as roughly 50% of the vulnerability to addiction is believed to be genetic, so too is roughly 50% believed to be experiential. This should not be conceptualized as an 'either-or' situation. It is not a question of biology versus environment. Genetic and experiential factors operate together to produce the behavioral phenotype of addiction. Furthermore, substantial evidence exists that environmental and social factors can influence the neurobiological substrates of addiction, including those referable to the functioning of the brain's reward circuitry (fig. 1).

Contributions to Addiction Vulnerability at the Animal Level

Considerable research has been devoted to identifying individual characteristics that predict high vulnerability to drug-seeking behavior in animals, with considerable success. Notable work in this area has been published by Le Moal, Piazza, Simon and colleagues [108, 109] of the Université of Bordeaux II in France, by Redolat et al. [110], and by Everitt and colleagues [78] of the University of Cambridge in the UK. Among the individual characteristics that have been found to predict high vulnerability to drug-seeking behavior are high reactivity to stress, high novelty-induced locomotor activity, high novelty seeking and high trait impulsivity. Provocatively, transgenerational effects of stress on drug-seeking behavior have been found, the adult offspring of stressed mothers showing increased locomotor responses to novelty and increased propensity to self-administer addictive drugs [109].

Contributions to Addiction Vulnerability at the Human Level

A wide variety of individual characteristics that predict high vulnerability to drug addiction at the human level have also been identified. Among these are sensation seeking and novelty seeking [111, 112], trait impulsivity [113, 114], antisocial conduct disorder – especially in adolescence [115] –, depression – which confers a 6-fold increased risk for drug or alcohol addiction [116, 117] – and attention deficit/hyperactivity disorder [118, 119]. In addition (as noted above), Blum et al. [66, 67] and Comings and Blum [70] have proposed that a reward deficiency syndrome referable to functional hypoactivity of dopaminergic brain reward substrates contributes significantly to addiction vulnerability at the human level. Also, Koob et al. [120–122] have proposed that a lack of homeostatic reward regulation, again referable to aberrant functionality of dopaminergic brain reward substrates, contributes significantly to addiction vulnerability in humans. Some of these human vulnerability factors to addiction have been successfully modeled at the animal level [123].

Neurobiologically Measured Aberrations of Brain Reward Function as Addiction Vulnerability Factors

Volkow et al. [73, 75] have carried out positron emission tomography studies of dopaminergic function in brains of awake human subjects, using displacement of [^{11}C]raclopride as a measure of extracellular dopamine. They reported a noteworthy finding: that healthy adult male subjects with robust striatal dopamine levels experience the psychostimulant methylphenidate as displeasurable, while subjects with deficits in striatal dopamine experience methylphenidate as pleasurable. This is intensely interesting and provocative, as the nucleus accumbens reward-relevant brain locus is located in the ventral striatum. Such findings suggest that striatal dopamine deficiency may constitute a vulnerability factor in addiction, which is conceptually congruent with Blum's [66, 67, 70] formulation of reward deficiency as an addiction risk factor.

Using positron emission tomography and displacement of [^{18}F]fluoroclebopride as a measure of extracellular dopamine in monkeys, Nader and colleagues [77] have reported provocative findings linking striatal dopamine, social rank within monkey troops, addictive drug exposure and vulnerability to addiction. This is extremely important work as it explicates the biopsychosocial model of addiction with undeniably

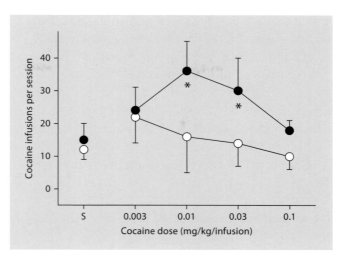

Fig. 5. Rank in a social hierarchy contributes to brain dopamine deficiency and vulnerability to addictive drug-taking behavior. S = Saline. * Significantly different from dominant monkeys at indicated dose, and from saline point, both at p < 0.05. ○ = Dominant monkeys; ● = submissive monkeys. Adapted from Morgan et al. [77].

robust neurobiological measures of functionality within the brain's reward circuitry. First, Nader and colleagues [77] found that individually housed, socially dominant monkeys show more robust levels of striatal dopamine than individually housed, socially submissive monkeys, raising the possibility that the submissive animals may have an increased risk for drug-seeking behavior. Second, they found that these differences in striatal dopamine levels between dominant and submissive monkeys were accentuated in socially housed monkeys. Third, they found that the submissive monkeys were, in fact, more drug seeking and drug taking, showing a robust elevation in the dose-response curve for self-administered cocaine (fig. 5).

Thus, submissiveness in a social hierarchy is correlated with dopamine deficiency in the reward circuitry of the brain, and both are correlated with enhanced drug-seeking and drug-taking behavior. To the same point, Robbins and colleagues [124] have shown that isolation rearing of rats impairs the reinforcing efficacy of intravenous cocaine and intra-accumbens amphetamine. Nader et al. [125] have also shown pronounced striatal dopamine deficiencies in cocaine-experienced monkeys as compared to cocaine-naive monkeys. Other workers, using positron emission tomography and displacement of $[^{11}C]$raclopride as a measure of extracellular striatal dopamine in both cats and monkeys, have similarly shown dopamine deficiencies in amphetamine-experienced animals as compared to amphetamine-naive animals [126, 127].

Additionally, Everitt and colleagues [78] have shown reduced dopamine D_2/D_3 receptor binding in nucleus accumbens of drug-naive, trait-impulsive laboratory rats. Relating this to addiction vulnerability, these researchers have shown that the highly impulsive rats are significantly more drug seeking than the nonimpulsive rats [78, 128]. Furthermore, Everitt and colleagues [129] have shown that high reactivity to novelty predicts the propensity to initiate drug self-administration, while high impulsivity predicts the propensity to progress from simple drug-taking behavior to addiction-like drug-taking behavior, characterized by persistent and compulsive drug taking in the face of aversive consequences.

This body of work is remarkable for tying together behavioral traits (impulsivity, high reactivity to novelty), social factors (dominance vs. submission), prior drug experience (cocaine or amphetamine exposure vs. nonexposure), dopamine functionality within the brain's reward circuitry (measured by dopamine displacement studies) and drug-seeking behavior. The biopsychosocial model of addiction seems well supported by such work, using laboratory animal models.

The Natural Progression of the Disease of Addiction

The disease of addiction is characterized by progressive stages. It always starts with occasional reward-driven use, which then progresses to steady (albeit nonaddictive) reward-driven use [130–132]. Reward-driven use progresses to habit-driven use, and habit-driven use progresses to compulsive use [24, 133–136]. At the human level, there is often psychological denial of aberrant or self-damaging behavior [137] coupled with impaired insight [138], often lasting for years. Addictive, abusive, self-damaging drug use coupled with psychological denial is then, for some addicts, followed by 'bottoming out' (loss of spouse, family, employment, home, car, possessions). For a fortunate subset of addicts, this is followed by treatment and achievement of abstinence. However, in most cases there is persistent vulnerability to drug craving and persistent vulnerability to relapse to drug-seeking behavior [134, 139–141].

Although the neurobiological substrates of the various stages of disease progression are not fully understood, Robbins and Everitt [142] have proposed that the progression of addiction from reward-driven behavior to habit-driven behavior correlates with a progression of the controlling neurobiological locus of the disease from the ventral striatum (nucleus accumbens) to the dorsal striatum. They base their hypothesis on several factors: the involvement of the dorsal striatum in habit formation, the phenomenon of pavlovian-to-instrumental transfer, and the existence of an anatomic ascending spiral of striato-nigral-striato loop pathways from the nucleus accumbens shell to the dorsolateral striatum. The first factor – involvement of the dorsal striatum in stimulus-response associations or habits – has long been recognized [143]. The second factor – pavlovian-to-instrumental transfer – is a learning phenomenon that sheds light on the interrelationships between the reward circuitry of the brain, habit learning and addictive behavior. In pavlovian-to-instrumental transfer, animals are first trained to associate a conditioned stimulus with a reward (pavlovian learning). The animals are then trained to perform an instrumental task (e.g. pressing a wall-mounted lever in their test chambers) to receive the same reward (instrumental learning). The animals are then exposed to extinction of the instrumental learning (i.e. the instrumental response is no longer rewarded). Presentation of the conditioned stimulus enhances instrumental responding during extinction, thus modeling an important component of addictive behavior (i.e. the ability of drug-associated environmental cues to drive drug-seeking behavior in the absence of drug-induced reward). Provocatively, lesions of the nucleus accumbens core and the central nucleus of the amygdala abolish pavlovian-to-instrumental transfer, while lesions of the nucleus accumbens shell and the basolateral amygdala have no effect [142]. Pharmacologically, dopamine D_2/D_3 receptor antagonism abolishes pavlovian-to-instrumental transfer, while dopamine agonists potentiate it [142]. The third factor – an ascending spiral of striato-nigral-striato loop pathways from the nucleus accumbens shell to the dorsolateral striatum – has been demonstrated anatomically by Haber et al. [144].

Putting all of these factors together, Robbins and Everitt [142] propose the following:

Compulsive drug-seeking behavior is inflexible, since it persists despite considerable cost to the addict, becomes dissociated from subjective measures of drug value, becomes elicited by specific environmental stimuli, and involves complex goal-directed behaviors for procurement and self-administration of drugs. Limbic cortical-ventral striatopallidal circuits that underlie goal-directed drug-seeking actions may eventually consolidate habitual, S-R [stimulus-response] drug seeking through engagement of corticostriatal loops operating through the dorsal striatum. This progression from action to habit may have its neural basis within the 'spiraling' loop circuitry of the striatum, by which each striatal domain regulates its own DA [dopaminergic] innervation and that of its adjacent domain in a ventral-to-dorsal progression [144]. Thus, the NAc [nucleus accumbens] shell regulates its own DA innervation via projections to the VTA [ventral tegmental area] and also that of the NAc core. The NAc core in turn regulates its own DA innervation via projections to the VTA and also that of the next, more dorsal tier of the dorsal striatum via projections to the substantia nigra pars compacta and so on. Chronically self-administered drugs, through their ability to increase striatal DA, may consolidate this ventral-to-dorsal striatal progression of control over drug-seeking as an habitual form of responding [142, 145].

This proposal is congruent both with neuroimaging studies [25, 146–148] and with electrophysiological studies [149].

Addiction and Physical Dependence – Different Phenomena and Different Brain Substrates

It is very important to realize that addiction and physical dependence are different phenomena with different underlying brain substrates [3]. Physical dependence results from the development of pharmacological tolerance, and manifests itself upon abrupt discontinuation of drug administration (or administration of an antagonist drug). Addiction is a chronic, progressively deteriorating disease characterized by compulsive drug use in the presence of harm to the addict and to the addict's life. Addiction is commonly described as the 'disease of the 5 Cs': *continued compulsive* drug use despite injurious *consequences,* coupled with loss of *control* and persistent drug *craving* [3].

Many drugs (including, but not limited to, antihypertensives, cardiac medications and asthma medications) produce pronounced physical dependence but are not addictive. Some drugs (e.g. cocaine) are highly addicting but produce little or no physical dependence. Furthermore, laboratory animals will avidly self-administer addictive drugs in the absence of tolerance, physical dependence or withdrawal discomfort [1, 3]. Indeed, laboratory animals will avidly self-administer addictive drugs in the absence of any prior drug exposure whatsoever, rendering the issue of self-administration due to physical dependence moot. The importance of this fact can hardly be overstated as it unambiguously shows that drug-taking behavior cannot simply be explained by the ability of addictive drugs to ameliorate the withdrawal discomfort associated with abstinence from prior administration of such drugs [1, 3].

Critically, the brain sites mediating volitional drug self-administration are different from those mediating the development and expression of physical dependence. This dissociation of brain substrates and loci subserving addiction and physical dependence was first demonstrated by Bozarth and Wise [150] in a pioneering and now classic series of experiments using direct intracerebral microinjections of opiates into specific brain loci in awake behaving animals. They found that laboratory rats willingly (indeed, avidly) self-administered opiates to the brain's reward loci, but that such self-administration (even if prolonged) does not evoke opiate physical dependence. Conversely, they found that opiate microinjection into more posterior brain stem loci (in the vicinity of the dorsal raphe nucleus) produces strong opiate physical dependence (and strong physical withdrawal symptoms upon abrupt discontinuation), but that animals do not self-administer opiates to those loci. This double dissociation of brain loci is definitive with respect to addiction and physical dependence being different phenomena.

Equally importantly, the different brain sites mediating volitional drug self-administration and physical dependence are, in turn, different from those mediating the antinociceptive properties of opiates. This additional dissociation of brain substrates and loci was first demonstrated by Pert and Yaksh [151] in an equally pioneering and now classic series of experiments using direct intracerebral microinjections of opiates into specific brain loci of awake behaving monkeys. The monkeys were fitted with an electrical plate on one foot, through which painful electrical stimulation was given. Each monkey had a manipulandum (a lever mounted on the front of its primate test chair) that it could depress to lower the intensity of the painful stimulation. Each monkey also had many surgically implanted intracerebral cannulae, through which morphine could be microinjected by the researchers. Hundreds of brain loci were tested for their ability to induce analgesia to the painful foot shock. Only two analgesic loci were found. One corresponded to the periaqueductal gray matter of the brain stem, and the second was in the vicinity of the lateral neospinothalamic pathway as it ascends through the lateral midbrain and into the periventricular and intralaminar nuclei of the thalamus [151]. From these brain loci, especially the periaqueductal gray area, descending neuronal tracts run down the spinal cord to synapse within the dorsal horns in order to activate synaptic pain gates [152–154], blocking ascending nociceptive neural signals and producing analgesia.

Thus, a triple dissociation manifests itself. The brain loci mediating opiate-seeking behavior are distinct from those mediating opiate-induced physical dependence, which are in turn distinct from those mediating opiate-induced analgesia. Further discussion of brain mechanisms and analgesia – and the false notion that medically appropriate opiate analgesia can induce opiate addiction – will be addressed below.

Persistent Drug Craving and Relapse – The Real Clinical Problem in Addiction

Any cigarette smoker who has tried to quit the smoking habit knows that the real clinical problem in addiction is persistent drug craving and relapse. As Mark Twain (Samuel Clemens), the famous 19th-century American author and humorist, phrased it: 'It's easy to quit smoking. I've done it hundreds of times'. Behind this amusing aphorism is a terrible truth: it is extremely difficult to overcome the persistent drug cravings that the abstinent addict is left with after having achieved (often with great difficulty) abstinence. This is why acute 'detoxification' programs are almost invariably clinical failures in treating drug addiction. Indeed, the failure rate is so high that physicians running such programs may be reasonably said to be engaging in medical malpractice.

Since the founding of the Alcoholics Anonymous organization in the 1930s and the publication of its so-called 'Big Book' [155], it has been recognized that there are three classical triggers to drug craving (and relapse to drug-seeking behavior) in recovering drug addicts: reexposure to drug, exposure to stress and reexposure to environmental cues previously associated with drinking or drugging.

In recent decades, the development of animal models of relapse have permitted a remarkable amount of research to be carried out on the neural substrates of craving and relapse. The first such model is the so-called 'reinstatement' model [46, 156, 157]. This model is built upon the intravenous drug self-administration animal model in which animals are intravenously catheterized and allowed to voluntarily self-administer addictive drugs. To model relapse, the animals are first allowed to self-administer a drug until highly stable day-to-day drug-taking behavior is achieved. Then, the addictive drug is removed from the infusion pump and saline (or vehicle) is substituted. The drug-taking behavior extinguishes due to lack of reinforcement. The animal is then tested daily until highly stable day-to-day nonresponding is achieved. Then, the animal is exposed to relapse triggers (drug, stress, cues) and the amount of drug-seeking responding (on the manipulandum which has previously activated the infusion pump and delivered the addictive drug) is measured, such responses not being reinforced by the drug. A second relapse model is the so-called 'reactivation' model [45, 46, 158], which is built upon the conditioned place preference animal model of drug-seeking behavior (see above).

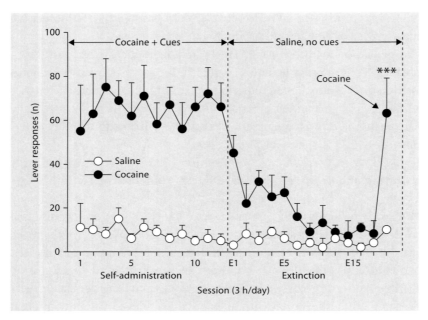

Fig. 6. Time-line graph of reinstatement (relapse) to addictive drug-seeking behavior. Means ± SEM. *** Significantly different from last extinction day at p < 0.001.

To model relapse in this model, the animal is allowed to acquire a conditioned place preference to an addictive drug. Then the animal is repeatedly exposed to the conditioned place preference test chamber (with open access to all compartments), day after day, until the drug-induced place preference is fully extinguished. Then, on the test day, the animal is exposed to relapse triggers, and the amount of drug-seeking behavior is measured as the amount of time spent in the previously drug-paired compartment. Both of these models yield remarkably robust relapse to drug-seeking behavior with seemingly high face, construct and predictive validity for human relapse (fig. 6) [159, 160].

Neuroanatomy and Neurochemistry of Brain Circuits Mediating Relapse

By a variety of research stratagems – including combining intracerebral microinjections or anatomically discrete intracerebral lesions with one of the animal relapse models outlined above – it has been possible to discover the brain circuits underlying relapse to drug-seeking behavior triggered by the three classical relapse triggers. Relapse to drug-seeking behavior triggered by noncontingent reexposure to a drug is mediated by the dopaminergic medial forebrain bundle tract linking the ventral tegmental area with the nucleus accumbens [46, 156, 157, 161].

Relapse to drug-seeking behavior triggered by stress appears to involve two separate neural circuits in the brain. The first circuit originates in the lateral-tegmental noradrenergic cell groups (especially nucleus A2, as described by Moore and Bloom [162]) and projects anteriorly to synapse in the hypothalamus, nucleus accumbens, amygdala and bed nucleus of the stria terminalis [156, 157, 161]. This relapse circuit uses norepinephrine as its major neurotransmitter. In view of the major role that the noradrenergic locus ceruleus plays in brain-mediated stress events [163], it is somewhat counterintuitive that the A2 lateral-tegmental nucleus, rather than the locus ceruleus, should be the major noradrenergic brain locus mediating stress-triggered relapse to drug-seeking behavior, but this seems to be the case. The second neural circuit mediating stress-triggered relapse to drug-seeking behavior originates in the central nucleus of the amygdala and projects to the bed nucleus of the stria terminalis. This neural circuit uses corticotrophin-releasing factor (CRF) as its major neurotransmitter.

Relapse to drug-seeking behavior triggered by environmental cues previously paired with drinking or drugging also appears to involve two separate neural circuits in the brain, one originating in the ventral subiculum of the hippocampus, and one originating in the basolateral complex of the amygdala. Both of these circuits use glutamate as their major neurotransmitter. In a pioneering series of experiments, Gardner and colleagues [164, 165] showed that discrete low-level electrical stimulation of these circuits triggers relapse to drug-seeking behavior, and demonstrated that these relapse circuits are glutamatergically mediated.

Knowing the exact neural circuits involved in mediating relapse to drug-seeking behavior, and their respective neurotransmitters, opens up the distinct possibility of being able to develop anticraving and antirelapse medication using medication development strategies that are highly targeted on specific neurobiological substrates of relapse [166–168].

Incubation of Craving – An Animal Model of the Extreme Fragility of Control over Vulnerability to Relapse in Human Addicts

In 2001, Grimm et al. [169] described a compelling phenomenon at the laboratory animal level, namely that relapse vulnerability to drug-seeking behavior incubates (grows more intense) with the mere passage of time. In this 'incubation of craving' model, animals are allowed to self-acquire the intravenous drug-taking habit. Once stable drug-taking is established, the animals are returned to their home cages, where they simply wait for varying amounts of time (days, weeks, months). Importantly, nothing is done to the animals during this waiting period. They are neither reexposed to the drug nor to stress nor to any drug-associated environmental cues, nor are they exposed to deliberate extinction of the drug-taking habit. Then, on the test day, they are returned to the test chamber in which they originally acquired the drug-taking

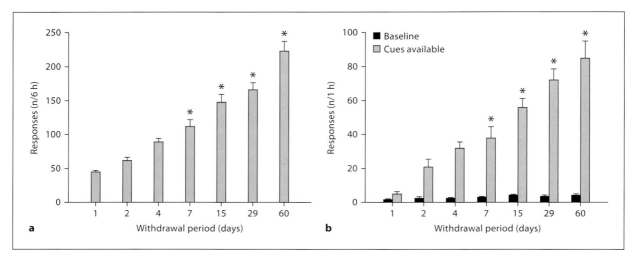

Fig. 7. Incubation (enhancement) of drug-craving with the mere passage of time. Drug-seeking behavior measured as extinction responding (**a**) and as cue-triggered relapse to drug-seeking behavior (**b**). From Grimm et al. [169]. *Significantly different from withdrawal day 1 at p < 0.01.

habit, and allowed access to the manipulandum (typically a wall-mounted lever or a nose poke detector device) that originally activated the infusion pump to deliver the drug. They are then tested for drug-seeking behavior (lever pressing, nose poking) in the absence (extinction testing) or presence (cue-triggered testing) of the environmental cues originally associated with the drug-taking behavior. Remarkably, a time-dependent increase ('incubation') in the intensity of drug-seeking behavior – whether measured as extinction responding or cue-triggered responding – is observed. After 4 days, drug-seeking behavior is approximately 100% greater than after 1 day. After 15 days, drug-seeking behavior is approximately 200% greater than after 1 day. After 60 days, drug-seeking behavior is approximately 400% greater than after 1 day. This remarkable increase in vulnerability to relapse to drug-seeking behavior with the mere passage of time is considered to be an animal model of the extreme fragility of control over relapse vulnerability, and the increase in this vulnerability with the passage of time that is so frequently reported by human addicts (fig. 7).

The same researchers subsequently found that this incubation of craving phenomenon corresponds to a postcocaine time-dependent increase in brain-derived neurotrophic factor (BDNF) protein levels within the mesolimbic dopaminergic reward and relapse circuits, specifically in the nucleus accumbens and amygdala [170]. This research group also explored the role of the amygdaloid extracellular signal-regulated kinase (ERK) signaling pathway in this incubation [171]. Cocaine seeking induced by exposure to cocaine cues was substantially higher after 30 days of cocaine withdrawal than after 1 day. Exposure to these cues increased ERK phosphorylation in the central, but not the basolateral, amygdala after 30 days of cocaine withdrawal, but not after 1 day. After 30 days of incubation of cocaine craving, inhibition of central (but not basolateral) amygdaloid ERK phosphorylation produced an inhibition of cocaine-seeking behavior. After 1 day of withdrawal, stimulation of central amygdaloid ERK phosphorylation increased cocaine-seeking behavior. All of this suggests that incubation of cocaine craving is mediated by time-dependent increases in the responsiveness of the central amygdaloid ERK pathway to cocaine cues. Central amygdaloid glutamate is also involved [172]. Central amygdala injections of the glutamate mGluR2/3 agonist LY379268 (which decreases glutamate release) attenuated the augmented cue-triggered drug-seeking behavior seen after 21 days of incubation, but had no effect after only 3 days of incubation. As the amygdala is critical to cue-triggered relapse [165], and the nucleus accumbens to drug- and stress-triggered relapse [156, 157, 161, 173], these findings are important.

They are especially important in the context of synaptic remodeling. Addiction obviously involves learning (stimulus-reward learning being an important substrate in the acquisition of addiction, stimulus-response learning being an important substrate in relapse responding). Beginning with the pioneering neuropsychological work by Hebb [174] in the 1940s, it has been widely appreciated that the neural substrate of learning must involve synaptic remodeling. In recent decades, it has come to be appreciated that two important mechanistic substrates of synaptic remodeling are long-term potentiation and long-term depression (LTD) [175]. Long-term potentiation and LTD have been demonstrated to be produced by addictive drugs in precisely those brain loci implicated in reward and relapse: the nucleus accumbens [176–179], amygdala [180, 181] and hippocampus [182–184]. As a neuronal trophic factor, BDNF may be involved in – may indeed be an underlying mechanism for – the synaptic remodeling in the nucleus accumbens, amygdala and hippocampus that may underlie the incubation of craving phenomenon and, by extension, the development of increased vulnerability to relapse among human addicts. Furthermore, such synaptic remodeling may underlie the very transition to the unregulated and compulsive drug-seeking behavior that characterizes addiction, inasmuch as this transition is associated with impaired glutamate receptor-dependent brain LTD [185]. If this be true, an entirely new strategy for antiaddiction, anticraving and antirelapse medication development could emerge, with medications that target BDNF-mediated synaptic remodeling in the nucleus accumbens, amygdala and hippocampus. Of course, such medication development need not be exclusive of anticraving and antirelapse medication development predicated on other neural mechanistic strategies, e.g. glutamate mGluR2/3 agonists [172] or selective dopamine D_3 receptor antagonists [83, 84, 186].

The Disentanglement of Important Addiction-Related Phenomena

From all of the above, it may be appreciated that a number of important phenomena are often confused, even among medical and other professionals who deal routinely with drug addiction and with patients impacted by it. It is important to disentangle these phenomena.

First, abusive drug-taking behavior is initially reward driven (the drug-induced high), and is directly referable to drug-induced activation of the ventral tegmental area-nucleus accumbens reward circuitry.

Second, abusive drug-seeking and drug-taking behavior becomes, with time, habit driven rather than reward driven. This transition arguably defines the onset of addictive drug-seeking behavior, and is arguably referable to a transition of the neural locus of control over drug-seeking behavior from the ventral tegmental-ventral neostriatal axis (medial ventral tegmental area and nucleus accumbens) to a more dorsolateral overlying set of neural loop circuits (involving the substantia nigra and dorsolateral neostriatum).

Third, addiction and physical dependence are different phenomena, the first referable to the forebrain mesolimbic and mesostriatal reward-related and habit-related circuitry, the second referable to neural loci in the vicinity of the midbrain dorsal raphe nucleus and the dorsal mesencephalon. Some drugs are addictive without producing physical dependence; other drugs produce physical dependence without being addictive.

Fourth, opiate- and cannabinoid-induced analgesia are distinct phenomena having nothing to do with opiate-induced or cannabinoid-induced addictive drug-taking behavior. Opiate-induced analgesia is referable to action on neural mechanisms on peripheral nociceptive neurons, spinal cord dorsal horn pain gates, dorsal root ganglia, brain stem tegmental spinothalamic and neospinothalamic pain relay nuclei, and the periaqueductal gray matter of the brain stem. Cannabinoid-induced analgesia is referable to action on neural mechanisms on peripheral nociceptive neurons, spinal cord dorsal horn pain gates, dorsal root ganglia and brain stem tegmental spinothalamic and neospinothalamic pain relay nuclei. Importantly, appropriate medical use of opiates or cannabinoids for the treatment of pain carries an extremely low risk of inducing addiction (see further discussion below).

Can One Induce Addiction by Long-Term Treatment of Pain with Opiates?

Far too many physicians and other health care professionals have uncritically accepted the false allegation that opiate addiction can be induced by medically appropriate long-term treatment of pain with opiates [186]. This leads to medical malpractice and the ethically unacceptable undertreatment of pain in millions of suffering patients. Equally unacceptably, this misconception permeates the law enforcement, judicial and legislative branches of government, with many egregious consequences. It also permeates ordinary society, causing many pain patients to refuse medically appropriate (indeed often essential) treatment of pain, with often horrible consequences for quality of life.

The truth of the matter is that although some chronic pain patients are at risk for addiction, they are a very small percentage of the total number of chronic pain patients. Reliable evidence exists to support the contention that appropriate medical treatment of pain with opiates does not incur a risk of addiction in the vast majority of pain patients. First, chronic pain inhibits opiate-seeking behavior in animal models [186, 187]. Second, chronic pain inhibits opiate-enhanced dopamine in the ventral tegmental area-nucleus accumbens reward/relapse neural circuitry [186, 188]. Third, chronic pain inhibits reward signaling through the ventral tegmental area-nucleus accumbens reward circuitry, as assessed using the electrical brain stimulation reward animal model [186, 189]. Fourth, chronic pain inhibits the development of opiate-induced physical dependence [186, 190]. These preclinical animal model and neurobiological data – together with an impressive corpus of human clinical data – has prompted the World Health Organization to issue the following guideline on the treatment of chronic pain: 'When opioids are used – even at heroic doses – in the appropriate medical control of chronic pain, addiction and drug abuse are not a major concern' [191].

Brain Reward/Antireward Pathways and Mechanism-Based Medication Development for Treatment of Addiction

At present, a number of effective pharmacotherapies exist for the treatment of drug addiction. The opiate agonist methadone has been shown to be effective in opiate addiction [192, 193], as has the partial opiate agonist buprenorphine [192–194]. Even heroin itself has been successfully used as a maintenance pharmacotherapy for opiate addiction [195]. Although the short half-life of heroin makes it a less than optimal choice for maintenance therapy for many patients, there appears to be a subset of opiate addicts who do better on heroin maintenance than on other opioid agonist therapies [195]. For highly motivated individuals with a strong desire to achieve abstinence from the opiate-taking habit, the long-acting opiate antagonist naltrexone has proven effective [193, 196].

Naltrexone has also proven to be effective for some alcoholics wishing to quell alcohol cravings [196–198]. The reason for the effectiveness of naltrexone in alcoholism is not clearly understood but may relate to the fact that the dopaminergic reward circuitry of the brain is heavily innervated by endogenous opioid peptide (endorphin and enkephalin) circuits, and this opioid peptidergic innervation is known to modulate the reward-enhancing properties of alcohol [199–201] and other addictive compounds (e.g. Δ^9-tetrahydrocannabinol, the addictive constituent in marijuana and hashish [202–204]).

Acamprosate is also claimed to have effectiveness against alcohol addiction [205], as is the $GABA_B$ receptor agonist baclofen [206–208]. The underlying mechanisms for acamprosate's putative effectiveness appear to involve re-normalization of alcohol-perturbed glutamatergic neurotransmission [209]. The underlying mechanisms for the effectiveness of baclofen are not fully clear, but its presumptive effectiveness at the human level is amply and well supported by many years of work with baclofen in preclinical animal models of addiction by Roberts and colleagues [210–215]. This work with baclofen in preclinical animal models of addiction suggests a broad potential clinical efficacy for baclofen in treating addiction at the human level, but thus far only preliminary studies on human patients have been undertaken with baclofen [208].

The acetylcholine nicotinic $\alpha_4\beta_2$-receptor partial agonist/α_7-receptor full agonist varenicline is clearly effective in treating nicotine addiction at the human level [216, 217]. Furthermore, varenicline appears superior to other treatments; the 1-year continuous abstinence rate from tobacco use is 23% for varenicline, as compared to 15% for bupropion and 10% for placebo [216]. The effectiveness of varenicline appears to be due to its action at the nicotinic $\alpha_4\beta_2$-receptor subtype; its action at the α_7-receptor subtype appears irrelevant to its efficacy [218]. Nicotine replacement therapy (e.g. the nicotine patch) is also effective in some patients for smoking cessation. Bupropion also appears to have efficacy in treating nicotine addiction [219], which may be partly due to its action as a dopamine reuptake inhibitor [220], and partly due to its action as a nicotinic receptor antagonist [221].

Yet, none of the above-listed pharmacotherapies is effective for a majority of the patients for whom the therapy should produce clinical benefit, and with the possible exception of baclofen, none of the above therapies is broadly effective against multidrug addiction.

Thus, there is a real need for further medication development in the field of addiction medicine. Fortunately, by reference to current knowledge of the involvement of brain reward/antireward pathways and substrates in addiction, mechanism-based medication development for the treatment of addiction is both rational and practical.

The fact that cocaine and other psychostimulants derive their addictive efficacies from inhibiting the synaptic reuptake of dopamine or by causing presynaptic release of dopamine in the reward-related and relapse-related nucleus accumbens makes the development of slow-onset long-acting dopamine transporter inhibitors for the treatment of psychostimulant addiction rational [222–226].

The fact that inhibition of medium spiny GABAergic neurons in the nucleus accumbens may constitute a final common pathway for addictive-drug-induced reward [227] makes development of GABAergic agonist therapies rational. As noted above, extraordinary promise has been seen with the $GABA_B$ receptor agonist baclofen in preclinical animal models [210–215], with some supporting evidence from preliminary human use [206–208]. Similarly, considerable promise has been seen with the indirect GABA agonist γ-vinyl GABA in preclinical animal models [228–237], again with some supporting evidence from preliminary human trials [238].

The fact that cannabinoids activate, and endocannabinoids mediate, brain reward and brain relapse circuits and substrates [202, 203, 205, 239–247] provides a mechanistic rationale for the development of cannabinoid CB$_1$ receptor antagonists as antiaddiction medications [40, 248–252].

The facts that glutamate circuits innervate and modulate brain reward mechanisms [253–260], and that glutamatergic circuits mediate at least some forms of relapse to drug-seeking behavior [164, 165], make the development of drugs acting on the glutamate circuitry of the brain attractive as potential antiaddiction medications [41, 261–265].

The fact that CRF is the neurotransmitter of one of the stress-triggered relapse circuits in the brain makes the development of anti-CRF medications attractive [167, 266–278].

A Final Comment

Addiction medicine has made enormous strides in recent decades. Arguably, addiction medicine has animal models with face validity, predictive validity and construct validity that are as good as or better than animal models in other medical specialties. More has been learned in the last few decades about the neurobiology of addiction, craving and relapse than would have been thought possible when Olds and Milner [6] first described the reward circuits of the brain in 1954. These tremendous advances in knowledge bode well for the development of definitive therapies for an illness that is as old as recorded human history.

Acknowledgments

The author is indebted to Ms. Stacey Saunders for editorial assistance, and to Dr. Zheng-Xiong Xi for assistance with the figures.

References

1 Gardner EL: Brain reward mechanisms; in Lowinson JH, Ruiz P, Millman RB, Langrod JG (eds): Substance Abuse. A Comprehensive Textbook, ed 4. Philadelphia, Lippincott Williams & Wilkins, 2005, pp 48–97.

2 Gardner EL: What we have learned about addiction from animal models of drug self-administration. Am J Addict 2000;9:285–313.

3 O'Brien CP, Gardner EL: Critical assessment of how to study addiction and its treatment: human and non-human animal models. Pharmacol Ther 2005; 108:18–58.

4 Gardner EL, David J: The neurobiology of chemical addiction; in Elster J, Skog OJ (eds): Getting Hooked. Rationality and the Addictions. Cambridge, Cambridge University Press, 1999, pp 93–136.

5 Wise RA, Gardner EL: Functional anatomy of substance-related disorders; in D'Haenen H, den Boer JA, Willner P (eds): Biological Psychiatry. New York, Wiley, 2002, pp 509–522.

6 Olds J, Milner P: Positive reinforcement produced by electrical stimulation of septal area and other regions of rat brain. J Comp Physiol Psychol 1954;47: 419–427.

7 Olds J: Pleasure centers in the brain. Sci Am 1956;95: 105–116.

8 Olds J: Hypothalamic substrates of reward. Physiol Rev 1962;42:554–604.

9 Olds ME, Olds J: Approach-avoidance analysis of rat diencephalon. J Comp Neurol 1963;120: 259–295.

10 Olds ME, Olds J: Drives, rewards and the brain; in Newcomb TM (ed): New Directions in Psychology. New York, Holt, Rinehart & Winston, 1965, pp 329–410.

11 Routtenberg A, Gardner EL, Huang YH: Self-stimulation pathways in the monkey, *Macaca mulatta*. Exp Neurol 1971;33:213–224.

12 Gallistel CR, Shizgal P, Yeomans JS: A portrait of the substrate for self-stimulation. Psychol Rev 1981;88:228–273.

13 Wise RA, Bozarth MA: Brain reward circuitry: four circuit elements 'wired' in apparent series. Brain Res Bull 1984;12:203–208.

14 Stuber GD, van Leeuwen WA, Sparta DR, Zhang F, Deisseroth K, Bonci A: Optogenetic control of brain reward circuitry. Paper presented at meetings of the Society for Neuroscience, Chicago, 2009 (abstract No. 686.8). 2009 Abstract Viewer/Itinerary Planner CD-ROM, Thirty-Ninth Annual Meeting of the Society for Neuroscience, Chicago, 2009. Washington, Society for Neuroscience, 2009.

15 Alheid GF, Heimer L: New perspectives in basal forebrain organization of special relevance for neuropsychiatric disorders: the striatopallidal, amygdaloid, and corticopetal components of substantia innominata. Neuroscience 1988;27:1–39.

16 Hubner CB, Koob GF: The ventral pallidum plays a role in mediating cocaine and heroin self-administration in the rat. Brain Res 1990;508:20–29.

17 Koob GF: Drugs of abuse: anatomy, pharmacology and function of reward pathways. Trends Pharmacol Sci 1992;13:177–184.

18 Kalivas PW, Churchill L, Klitenick MA: The circuitry mediating the translation of motivational stimuli into adaptive motor responses; in Kalivas PW, Barnes CD (eds): Limbic Motor Circuits and Neuropsychiatry. Boca Raton, CRC, 1993, pp 237–287.

19 Napier TC: Transmitter actions and interactions on pallidal neuronal function; in Kalivas PW, Barnes CD (eds): Limbic Motor Circuits and Neuropsychiatry. Boca Raton, CRC, 1993, pp 124–153.

20 Gong WH, Neill D, Justice JB Jr: Conditioned place preference and locomotor activation produced by injection of psychostimulants into ventral pallidum. Brain Res 1996;707:64–74.

21 Hasenöhrl RU, Frisch C, Huston JP: Evidence for anatomical specificity for the reinforcing effects of SP in the nucleus basalis magnocellularis region. Neuroreport 1998;9:7–10.

22 McBride WJ, Murphy JM, Ikemoto S: Localization of brain reinforcement mechanisms: intracranial self-administration and intracranial place-conditioning studies. Behav Brain Res 1999;101:129–152.

23 White NM, Milner PM: The psychobiology of reinforcers. Annu Rev Psychol 1992;43:443–471.

24 Robbins TW, Everitt BJ: Drug addiction: bad habits add up. Nature 1999;398:567–570.

25 Garavan H, Pankiewicz J, Bloom A, Cho J-K, Sperry L, Ross TJ, Salmeron BJ, Risinger R, Kelley D, Stein EA: Cue-induced cocaine craving: neuroanatomical specificity for drug users and drug stimuli. Am J Psychiatry 2000;157:1789–1798.

26 Higgins JW, Mahl GF, Delgado JMR, Hamlin H: Behavioral changes during intracerebral electrical stimulation. AMA Arch Neurol Psychiatry 1956;76:399–419.

27 Delgado JMR, Hamlin H: Spontaneous and evoked electrical seizures in animals and in humans; in Ramey ER, O'Doherty DS (eds): Electrical Studies on the Unanesthetized Brain. New York, Harper (Hoeber Medical Division), 1960, pp 133–158.

28 Heath RG, Mickle WH: Evaluation of seven years' experience with depth electrode studies in human patients; in Ramey ER, O'Doherty DS (eds): Electrical Studies on the Unanesthetized Brain. New York, Harper (Hoeber Medical Division), 1960, pp 214–247.

29 Sem-Jacobsen W, Torkildsen A: Depth recording and electrical stimulation in the human brain; in Ramey ER, O'Doherty DS (eds): Electrical Studies on the Unanesthetized Brain. New York, Harper (Hoeber Medical Division), 1960, pp 280–288.

30 Bishop MP, Elder ST, Heath RG: Intracranial self-stimulation in man. Science 1963;140:394–396.

31 Heath RG: Electrical self-stimulation of the brain in man. Am J Psychiatry 1963;120:571–577.

32 Stein L, Ray OS: Brain stimulation reward 'thresholds' self-determined in rat. Psychopharmacologia 1960;1:251–256.

33 Gardner EL: An improved technique for determining brain reward thresholds in primates. Behav Res Methods Instrum 1971;3:273–274.

34 Miliaressis E, Rompré P-P, Laviolette P, Philippe L, Coulombe D: The curve-shift paradigm in self-stimulation. Physiol Behav 1986;37:85–91.

35 Coulombe D, Miliaressis E: Fitting intracranial self-stimulation data with growth models. Behav Neurosci 1987;101:209–214.

36 Anthony JC, Warner LA, Kessler RC: Comparative epidemiology of dependence on tobacco, alcohol, controlled substances, and inhalants: basic findings from the National Comorbidity Survey. Exp Clin Psychol 1994;2:244–268.

37 Vorel SR, Ashby CR Jr, Paul M, Liu X, Hayes R, Hagan JJ, Middlemiss DN, Stemp G, Gardner EL: Dopamine D_3 receptor antagonism inhibits cocaine-seeking and cocaine-enhanced brain reward in rats. J Neurosci 2002;22:9595–9603.

38 Pak AC, Ashby CR Jr, Heidbreder CA, Pilla M, Gilbert J, Xi Z-X, Gardner EL: The selective dopamine D_3 receptor antagonist SB-277011A reduces nicotine-enhanced brain reward and nicotine-paired environmental cue functions. Int J Neuropsychopharmacol 2006;9:585–602.

39 Spiller K, Xi Z-X, Peng X-Q, Newman AH, Ashby CR Jr, Heidbreder CA, Gaál J, Gardner EL: The selective dopamine D_3 receptor antagonists SB-277011A and NGB 2904 and the putative partial D_3 receptor agonist BP-897 attenuate methamphetamine-enhanced brain-stimulation reward in rats. Psychopharmacology 2008;196: 533–542.

40 Xi Z-X, Spiller K, Pak AC, Gilbert J, Dillon C, Li X, Peng X-Q, Gardner EL: Cannabinoid CB1 receptor antagonists attenuate cocaine's rewarding effects: experiments with self-administration and brain-stimulation reward in rats. Neuropsychopharmacology 2008;33:1735–1745.

41 Li X, Li J, Peng X-Q, Spiller K, Gardner EL, Xi Z-X: Metabotropic glutamate receptor 7 modulates cocaine's rewarding effects in rats: involvement of a ventral pallidal GABAergic mechanism. Neuropsychopharmacology 2009;34:1783–1796.

42 Gardner EL, Lowinson JH: Drug craving and positive/negative hedonic brain substrates activated by addicting drugs. Semin Neurosci 1993;5:359–368.

43 Xi Z-X, Spiller K, Gardner EL: Cannabinoid CB1 and CB2 receptors modulate brain reward function in opposite directions in rats. Paper presented at meetings of the Society for Neuroscience, Chicago, 2009 (abstract No. 449.13). 2009 Abstract Viewer/Itinerary Planner CD-ROM, Thirty-Ninth Annual Meeting of the Society for Neuroscience, Chicago, 2009. Washington, Society for Neuroscience, 2009.

44 Tzschentke TM: Measuring reward with the conditioned place preference paradigm: a comprehensive review of drug effects, recent progress and new issues. Prog Neurobiol 1998;56:613–672.

45 Tzschentke TM: Measuring reward with the conditioned place preference (CPP) paradigm: update of the last decade. Addict Biol 2007;12:227–462.

46 Gardner EL, Wise RA: Animal models of addiction; in Charney DS, Nestler EJ (eds): Neurobiology of Mental Illness, ed 3. Oxford, Oxford University Press, 2009, pp 757–774.

47 Yokel RA, Wise RA: Increased lever pressing for amphetamine after pimozide in rats: implications for a dopamine theory of reward. Science 1975;187: 547–549.

48 Gardner EL, Chen J, Paredes W: Overview of chemical sampling techniques. J Neurosci Methods 1993; 48:173–197.

49 Wise RA: In vivo estimates of extracellular dopamine and dopamine metabolite levels during intravenous cocaine or heroin self-administration. Semin Neurosci 1993;5:337–342.

50 Wise RA, Leone P, Rivest R, Leeb K: Elevations of nucleus accumbens dopamine and DOPAC levels during intravenous heroin self-administration. Synapse 1995;21:140–148.

51 Wise RA, Newton P, Leeb K, Burnette B, Pocock D, Justice JB Jr: Fluctuations in nucleus accumbens dopamine concentration during intravenous cocaine self-administration in rats. Psychopharmacology 1995;120:10–20.

52 Solomon RL, Corbit JD: An opponent-process theory of motivation. 1. Temporal dynamics of affect. Psychol Rev 1974;81:119–145.

53 Solomon RL: The opponent-process theory of acquired motivation: the costs of pleasure and the benefits of pain. Am Psychologist 1980;35: 691–712.

54 Solomon RL: Recent experiments testing an opponent-process theory of acquired motivation. Acta Neurobiol Exp (Wars) 1980;40:271–289.

55 Koob GF, Stinus L, le Moal M, Bloom FE: Opponent process theory of motivation: neurobiological evidence from studies of opiate dependence. Neurosci Biobehav Rev 1989;13:135–140.

56 Koob GF, Caine SB, Parsons L, Markou A, Weiss F: Opponent process model and psychostimulant addiction. Pharmacol Biochem Behav 1997;57: 513–521.

57 Koob GF, le Moal M: Neurobiological mechanisms for opponent motivational processes in addiction. Philos Trans R Soc Lond B Biol Sci 2008;363: 3113–3123.

58 Nazzaro JM, Seeger TF, Gardner EL: Morphine differentially affects ventral tegmental and substantia nigra brain reward thresholds. Pharmacol Biochem Behav 1981;14:325–331.

59 Broderick PA, Gardner EL, van Praag HM: In vivo electrochemical evidence for a differential enkephalinergic modulation of dopamine in rat nigrostriatal and mesolimbic systems: correlated behavioral stereotypy results. Paper presented at meetings of the International Narcotic Research Conference, Garmisch-Partenkirchen, 1983.

60 Broderick PA, Gardner EL, van Praag HM: In vivo electrochemical and behavioral evidence for specific neural substrates modulated differentially by enkephalin in rat stimulant stereotypy and locomotion. Biol Psychiatry 1984;19:45–54.

61 Kokkinidis L, McCarter BD: Postcocaine depression and sensitization of brain-stimulation reward: analysis of reinforcement and performance effects. Pharmacol Biochem Behav 1990;36:463–471.

62 Markou A, Koob GF: Postcocaine anhedonia: an animal model of cocaine withdrawal. Neuropsychopharmacology 1991;4:17–26.

63 Schulteis G, Markou A, Cole M, Koob GF: Decreased brain reward produced by ethanol withdrawal. Proc Natl Acad Sci USA 1995;92:5880–5884.

64 Gardner EL, Lepore M: Withdrawal from a single small dose of marijuana elevates baseline brain-stimulation reward thresholds in rats. Paper presented at Winter Conference on Brain Research, Aspen, 1996.

65 Epping-Jordan MP, Watkins SS, Koob GF, Markou A: Dramatic decreases in brain reward function during nicotine withdrawal. Nature 1998;393: 76–79.

66 Blum K, Cull JG, Braverman ER, Comings DE: Reward deficiency syndrome. Am Sci 1996;84: 132–145.

67 Blum K, Sheridan PJ, Wood RC, Braverman ER, Chen TJH, Cull JG, Comings DE: The D_2 dopamine receptor gene as a determinant of reward deficiency syndrome. J R Soc Med 1996;89:396–400.

68 Gardner EL, Blum K: Neurobiology and genetics of addiction: implications of 'reward deficiency syndrome' for therapeutic strategies in chemical dependency. Paper presented at Russell Sage Foundation Conference on Addiction, New York, 1997.

69 Gardner EL: Neurobiology and genetics of addiction: implications of 'reward deficiency syndrome' for therapeutic strategies in chemical dependency; in Elster J (ed): Addiction. Entries and Exits. New York, Russell Sage Foundation, 1999, pp 57–119.

70 Comings DE, Blum K: Reward deficiency syndrome: genetic aspects of behavioral disorders. Prog Brain Res 2000;126:325–341.

71 Gardner EL: Reward behaviors as a function of hypo-dopaminergic activity: animal models of reward deficiency syndrome. Mol Psychiatry 2001; 6(suppl 1):S4.

72 Blum K, Noble EP, Sheridan PJ, Montgomery A, Ritchie T, Jadadeeswaran P, Nogami H, Briggs AH, Cohn JB: Allelic association of the human dopamine D_2 receptor gene in alcoholism. JAMA 1990;263: 2055–2059.

73 Volkow ND, Wang G-J, Fowler JS, Logan J, Gatley SJ, Gifford A, Hitzemann R, Ding Y-S, Pappas N: Prediction of reinforcing responses to psychostimulants in humans by brain dopamine D_2 receptor levels. Am J Psychiatry 1999;156:1440–1443.

74 Volkow ND, Fowler JS, Wang G-J, Ding Y-S, Gatley SJ: Role of dopamine in the therapeutic and reinforcing effects of methylphenidate in humans: results from imaging studies. Eur Neuropsychopharmacol 2002;12:557–566.

75 Volkow ND, Wang G-J, Fowler JS, Thanos PP, Logan J, Gatley SJ, Gifford A, Ding Y-S, Wong C, Pappas N: Brain DA D_2 receptors predict reinforcing effects of stimulants in humans: replication study. Synapse 2002;46:79–82.

76 Volkow ND, Wang G-J, Telang F, Fowler JS, Logan J, Jayne M, Ma Y, Pradhan K, Wong C: Profound decreases in dopamine release in striatum in detoxified alcoholics: possible orbitofrontal involvement. J Neurosci 2007;27:12700–12706.

77 Morgan D, Grant KA, Gage HD, Mach RH, Kaplan JR, Prioleau O, Nader SH, Buchheimer N, Ehrenkaufer RL, Nader MA: Social dominance in monkeys: dopamine D_2 receptors and cocaine self-administration. Nat Neurosci 2002;5:169–174.

78 Dalley JW, Fryer TD, Brichard L, Robinson ESJ, Theobald DEH, Lääne K, Peña Y, Murphy ER, Shah Y, Probst K, Abakumova I, Aigbirhio FI, Richards HK, Hong Y, Baron J-C, Everitt BJ, Robbins TW: Nucleus accumbens $D_{2/3}$ receptors predict trait impulsivity and cocaine reinforcement. Science 2007;315:1267–1270.

79 Staley JK, Mash DC: Adaptive increase in D_3 dopamine receptors in the brain reward circuits of human cocaine fatalities. J Neurosci 1996;16: 6100–6106.

80 Mash DC: Are neuroadaptations in D_3 dopamine receptors linked to the development of cocaine dependence? Mol Psychiatry 1997;2:7–8.

81 Gardner EL: Use of animal models to develop anti-addiction medications. Curr Psychiatry Rep 2008; 10:377–384.

82 Xi Z-X, Gardner EL: Hypothesis-driven medication discovery for the treatment of psychostimulant addiction. Curr Drug Abuse Rev 2008;1:303–327.

83 Xi Z-X, Spiller K, Gardner EL: Mechanism-based medication development for the treatment of nicotine dependence. Acta Pharmacol Sin 2009;30: 723–739.

84 Heidbreder CA, Gardner EL, Xi Z-X, Thanos PK, Mugnaini M, Hagan JJ, Ashby CR Jr: The role of central dopamine D_3 receptors in drug addiction: a review of pharmacological evidence. Brain Res Brain Res Rev 2005;49:77–105.

85 Heidbreder CA, Andreoli M, Marcon C, Hutcheson DM, Gardner EL, Ashby CR Jr: Evidence for the role of dopamine D_3 receptors in oral operant alcohol self-administration and reinstatement of alcohol-seeking behavior in mice. Addict Biol 2007;12:35–50.

86 Beitner-Johnson D, Guitart X, Nestler EJ: Dopaminergic brain reward regions of Lewis and Fischer rats display different levels of tyrosine hydroxylase and other morphine- and cocaine-regulated phosphoproteins. Brain Res 1991;561: 147–150.

87 Guitart X, Beitner-Johnson D, Marby DW, Kosten TA, Nestler EJ: Fischer and Lewis rat strains differ in basal levels of neurofilament proteins and their regulation by chronic morphine in the mesolimbic dopamine system. Synapse 1992;12:242–253.

88 Berrettini WH, Ferraro TN, Alexander RC, Buchberg AM, Vogel WH: Quantitative trait loci mapping of three loci controlling morphine preference using inbred mouse strains. Nat Genet 1994;7:54–58.

89 Crawley JN, Belknap JK, Collins A, Crabbe JC, Frankel W, Henderson N, Hitzemann RJ, Maxson SC, Miner LL, Silva AJ, Wehner JM, Wynshaw-Boris A, Paylor R: Behavioral phenotypes of inbred mouse strains: implications and recommendations for molecular studies. Psychopharmacology 1997;132: 107–124.

90 Brodkin ES, Carlezon WA Jr, Haile CN, Kosten TA, Heninger GR, Nestler EJ: Genetic analysis of behavioral, neuroendocrine, and biochemical parameters in inbred rodents: initial studies in Lewis and Fischer 344 rats and in A/J and C57BL/6J mice. Brain Res 1998;805:55–68.

91 McBride WJ, Li TK: Animal models of alcoholism: neurobiology of high alcohol-drinking behavior in rodents. Crit Rev Neurobiol 1998;12:339–369.

92 Crabbe JC, Phillips TJ, Buck KJ, Cunningham CL, Belknap JK: Identifying genes for alcohol and drug sensitivity: recent progress and future directions. Trends Neurosci 1999;22:173–179.

93 Nestler EJ: Genes and addiction. Nat Genet 2000; 26:277–281.

94 Dole VP, Nyswander M: A medical treatment for diacetylmorphine (heroin) addiction: a clinical trial with methadone hydrochloride. JAMA 1965;193: 646–650.

95 Dole VP, Nyswander ME, Kreek MJ: Narcotic blockade: a medical technique for stopping heroin use by addicts. Trans Assoc Am Physicians 1966;79: 122–136.

96 Wise RA: The dopamine synapse and the notion of 'pleasure centers' in the brain. Trends Neurosci 1980;3:91–95.

97 Lee R-S, Criado JE, Koob GF, Henriksen SJ: Cellular responses of nucleus accumbens neurons to opiate-seeking behavior. 1. Sustained responding during heroin self-administration. Synapse 1999;33:49–58.

98 Schultz W, Apicella P, Scarnati E, Ljungberg T: Neuronal activity in monkey ventral striatum related to the expectation of reward. J Neurosci 1992;12:4595–4610.

99 Chang J-Y, Sawyer SF, Lee R-S, Woodward DJ: Electrophysiological and pharmacological evidence for the role of the nucleus accumbens in cocaine self-administration in freely moving rats. J Neurosci 1994;14:1224–1244.

100 Kobayashi S, Schultz W: Influence of reward delays on responses of dopamine neurons. J Neurosci 2008; 28:7837–7846.

101 Gregorios-Pippas L, Tobler PN, Schultz W: Short-term temporal discounting of reward value in human ventral striatum. J Neurophysiol 2009;101: 1507–1523.

102 Hare TA, O'Doherty J, Camerer CF, Schultz W, Rangel A: Dissociating the role of the orbitalfrontal cortex and the striatum in the computation of goal values and prediction errors. J Neurosci 2008;28: 5623–5630.

103 Peoples LL, Uzwiak AJ, Gee F, Fabbricatore AT, Muccino KJ, Mohta BD, West MO: Phasic accumbal firing may contribute to the regulation of drug taking during intravenous cocaine self-administration sessions. Ann NY Acad Sci 1999;877:781–787.

104 Peoples LL, Cavanaugh D: Differential changes in signal and background firing of accumbal neurons during cocaine self-administration. J Neurophysiol 2003;90:993–1010.

105 Uhl GR: Molecular genetics of substance abuse vulnerability: remarkable recent convergence of genome scan results. Ann NY Acad Sci 2004;1025: 1–13.

106 Uhl GR, Drgan T, Johnson C, Fatusin OO, Liu Q-R, Contoreggi C, Li C-Y, Buck K, Crabbe J: 'Higher order' addiction molecular genetics: convergent data from genome-wide association in humans and mice. Biochem Pharmacol 2008;75:98–111.

107 Khokhar JY, Ferguson CS, Zhu AZX, Tyndale RF: Pharmacogenetics of drug dependence: role of gene variations in susceptibility and treatment. Annu Rev Pharmacol Toxicol 2010;50:39–61.

108 Piazza PV, Maccari S, Deminière JM, le Moal M, Mormède P, Simon H: Corticosterone levels determine individual vulnerability to amphetamine self-administration. Proc Natl Acad Sci USA 1991;88: 2088–2092.

109 Deminière JM, Piazza PV, Guegan G, Abrous N, Maccari S, le Moal M, Simon H: Increased locomotor response to novelty and propensity to intravenous amphetamine self-administration in adult offspring of stressed mothers. Brain Res 1992;586: 135–139.

110 Redolat R, Pérez-Martinez A, Carrasco MC, Mesa P: Individual differences in novelty-seeking and behavioral responses to nicotine: a review of animal studies. Curr Drug Abuse Rev 2009;2:230–242.

111 Sher KJ, Bartholow BD, Wood MD: Personality and substance use disorders: a prospective study. J Consult Clin Psychol 2000;68:818–829.

112 Zuckerman M, Kuhlman DM: Personality and risk-taking: common biosocial factors. J Pers 2000;68: 999–1029.

113 Mitchell SH: Measuring impulsivity and modeling its association with cigarette smoking. Behav Cogn Neurosci Rev 2004;3:261–275.

114 Perkins KA, Lerman C, Coddington SB, Jetton C, Karelitz JL, Scott JA, Wilson AS: Initial nicotine sensitivity in humans as a function of impulsivity. Psychopharmacology 2008;200:529–544.

115 Crowley TJ, Mikulich SK, Macdonald M, Young SE, Zerbe GO: Substance-dependent, conduct-disordered adolescent males: severity of diagnosis predicts 2-year outcome. Drug Alcohol Depend 1998;49:225–237.

116 Regier DA, Farmer ME, Rae DS, Locke BZ, Keith D, Judd LL, Goodwin FK: Comorbidity of mental disorders with alcohol and other drug abuse. JAMA 1990;264:2511–2518.

117 Kessler RC, Crum RM, Warner LA, Nelson CB, Schulenberg J, Anthony JC: Lifetime co-occurrence of DSM-III-R alcohol abuse and dependence with other psychiatric disorders in the National Comorbidity Survey. Arch Gen Psychiatry 1997;53: 232–240.

118 Wilson JJ, Levin FR: Attention deficit hyperactivity disorder (ADHD) and substance use disorders. Curr Psychiatry Rep 2001;3:497–506.

119 Wilens TE: Attention-deficit/hyperactivity disorder and the substance use disorders: the nature of the relationship, subtypes at risk, and treatment issues. Psychiatr Clin North Am 2004;27:283–301.

120 Koob GF, le Moal M: Drug addiction, dysregulation of reward, and allostasis. Neuropsychopharmacology 2001;24:97–129.

121 Koob GF, Ahmed SH, Boutrel B, Chen SA, Kenny PJ, Markou A, O'Dell LE, Parsons LH, Sanna PP: Neurobiological mechanisms in the transition from drug use to drug dependence. Neurosci Biobehav Rev 2004;27:739–749.

122 Koob GF: Hedonic homeostatic dysregulation as a driver of drug-seeking behavior. Drug Discov Today Dis Models 2008;5:207–215.

123 Lepore M, Vorel R, Gardner EL: Studies on the neurobiological interrelationship between vulnerability to depression and vulnerability to drug abuse in animal models. Behav Pharmacol 1995;6(suppl 1):82–84.

124 Phillips GD, Howes SR, Whitelaw RB, Robbins TW, Everitt BJ: Isolation rearing impairs the reinforcing efficacy of intravenous cocaine or intra-accumbens d-amphetamine: impaired response to intra-accumbens D_1 and D_2/D_3 dopamine receptor antagonists. Psychopharmacology 1994;115:419–429.

125 Nader MA, Morgan D, Gage HD, Nader SH, Calhoun TL, Buchheimer N, Ehrenkaufer R, Mach RH: PET imaging of dopamine D_2 receptors during chronic cocaine self-administration in monkeys. Nat Neurosci 2006;9:1050–1056.

126 Ginovart N, Farde L, Halldin C, Swahn CG: Changes in striatal D_2-receptor density following chronic treatment with amphetamine as assessed with PET in nonhuman primates. Synapse 1999;31:154–162.

127 Ginovart N, Wilson AA, Houle S, Kapur S: Amphetamine pretreatment induces a change in both D_2-receptor density and apparent affinity: a [^{11}C]raclopride positron emission tomography study in cats. Biol Psychiatry 2004;55:1188–1194.

128 Lee B, London ED, Poldrack RA, Farahi J, Nacca A, Monterosso JR, Mumford JA, Bokarius AV, Dahlbom M, Mukherjee J, Bilder RM, Brody AL, Mandelkern MA: Striatal dopamine D_2/D_3 receptor availability is reduced in methamphetamine dependence and is linked to impulsivity. J Neurosci 2009; 29:14734–14740.

129 Belin D, Mar AC, Dalley JW, Robbins TW, Everitt BJ: High impulsivity predicts the switch to compulsive cocaine-taking. Science 2008;320:1352–1355.

130 di Chiara G, Bassareo V, Fenu S, de Luca MA, Spina L, Cadoni C, Acquas E, Carboni E, Valentini V, Lecca D: Dopamine and drug addiction: the nucleus accumbens shell connection. Neuropharmacology 2004;47(suppl 1):227–241.

131 Wise RA: Dopamine, learning and motivation. Nat Rev Neurosci 2004;5:483–494.

132 Ikemoto S, Qin M, Liu Z-H: The functional divide for primary reinforcement of D-amphetamine lies between the medial and lateral ventral striatum: is the division of the nucleus accumbens core, shell, and olfactory tubercle valid? J Neurosci 2005;25: 5061–5065.

133 Tiffany ST: A cognitive model of drug urges and drug-use behavior: role of automatic and non-automatic processes. Psychol Rev 1990;97:146–168.

134 O'Brien CP, McLellan AT: Myths about the treatment of addiction. Lancet 1996;347:237–240.

135 Everitt BJ, Dickinson A, Robbins TW: The neuropsychological basis of addictive behaviour. Brain Res Rev 2001;36:129–138.

136 Everitt BJ, Robbins TW: Neural systems of reinforcement for drug addiction: from actions to habits to compulsion. Nat Neurosci 2005;8:1481–1489.

137 Verdejo-García A, Pérez-García M: Substance abusers' self-awareness of the neurobehavioral consequences of addiction. Psychiatry Res 2008;158: 172–180.

138 Goldstein R, Craig AD, Bechara A, Garavan H, Childress AR, Paulus MP, Volkow ND: The neurocircuitry of impaired insight in drug addiction. Trends Cogn Sci 2009;13:372–380.

139 Childress AR, Hole AV, Ehrman RN, Robbins SJ, McLellan AT, O'Brien CP: Cue reactivity and cue reactivity interventions in drug dependence. NIDA Res Monogr 1993;137:73–95.

140 Leshner AI: Addiction is a brain disease, and it matters. Science 1997;278:45–47.

141 O'Brien CP, Childress AR, Ehrman R, Robbins SJ: Conditioning factors in drug abuse: can they explain compulsion? J Psychopharmacol 1998;12: 15–22.

142 Robbins TW, Everitt BJ: Limbic-striatal memory systems and drug addiction. Neurobiol Learn Mem 2002;78:625–636.

143 White NM: Some highlights of research on the effects of caudate nucleus lesions over the past 200 years. Behav Brain Res 2009;199:3–23.

144 Haber SN, Fudge JL, McFarland NR: Striatonigrostriatal pathways in primates form an ascending spiral from the shell to the dorsolateral striatum. J Neurosci 2000;20:2369–2382.

145 Everitt BJ, Belin D, Economidou D, Pelloux Y, Dalley JW, Robbins TW: Neural mechanisms underlying the vulnerability to develop compulsive drug-seeking habits and addiction. Philos Trans R Soc Lond B Biol Sci 2008;363:3125–3135.

146 Letchworth SR, Nader MA, Smith HR, Friedman DP, Porrino LJ: Progression of changes in dopamine transporter binding site density as a result of cocaine self-administration in rhesus monkeys. J Neurosci 2001;21:2799–2807.

147 Porrino LJ, Daunais JB, Smith HR, Nader MA: The expanding effects of cocaine: studies in a nonhuman primate model of cocaine self-administration. Neurosci Biobehav Rev 2004;27:813–820.

148 Volkow ND, Wang G-J, Telang F, Fowler JS, Logan J, Childress AR, Jayne M, Ma YM, Wong C: Cocaine cues and dopamine in dorsal striatum: mechanism of craving in cocaine addiction. J Neurosci 2006;26: 6583–6588.

149 Takahashi Y, Roesch MR, Stalnaker TA, Schoenbaum G: Cocaine shifts the balance of associative encoding from ventral to dorsolateral striatum. Front Integr Neurosci 2007;1:11.

150 Bozarth MA, Wise RA: Anatomically distinct opiate receptor fields mediate reward and physical dependence. Science 1984;224:516–517.

151 Pert A, Yaksh T: Sites of morphine induced analgesia in the primate brain: relation to pain pathways. Brain Res 1974;80:135–140.

152 Melzack R, Wall PD: Pain mechanisms: a new theory. Science 1965;150:971–979.

153 Schaible HG: Peripheral and central mechanisms of pain generation. Handb Exp Pharmacol 2007;177: 3–28.

154 D'Mello R, Dickenson AH: Spinal cord mechanisms of pain. Br J Anaesth 2008;101:8–16.

155 Alcoholics Anonymous: Alcoholics Anonymous Big Book, ed 1. New York, Alcoholics Anonymous World Services, 1939.

156 Shalev U, Grimm JW, Shaham Y: Neurobiology of relapse to heroin and cocaine seeking: a review. Pharmacol Rev 2002;54:1–42.

157 Shaham Y, Shalev U, Lu L, de Wit H, Stewart J: The reinstatement model of drug relapse: history, methodology and major findings. Psychopharmacology 2003;168:3–20.

158 Aguilar MA, Rodríguez-Arias M, Miñarro J: Neurobiological mechanisms of the reinstatement of drug-conditioned place preference. Brain Res Rev 2009;59:253–277.

159 Epstein DH, Preston KL: The reinstatement model and relapse prevention: a clinical perspective. Psychopharmacology 2003;168:31–41.

160 Epstein DH, Preston KL, Stewart J, Shaham Y: Toward a model of drug relapse: an assessment of the validity of the reinstatement procedure. Psychopharmacology 2006;189:1–16.

161 Stewart J: Pathways to relapse: the neurobiology of drug- and stress-induced relapse to drug-taking. J Psychiatry Neurosci 2000;25:125–136.

162 Moore RY, Bloom FE: Central catecholamine neuron systems: anatomy and physiology of the norepinephrine and epinephrine systems. Annu Rev Neurosci 1979;2:113–168.

163 Itoi K: Ablation of the central noradrenergic neurons for unraveling their roles in stress and anxiety. Ann NY Acad Sci 2008;1129:47–54.

164 Vorel SR, Liu X, Hayes RJ, Spector JA, Gardner EL: Relapse to cocaine-seeking after hippocampal theta burst stimulation. Science 2001;292:1175–1178.

165 Hayes RJ, Vorel SR, Spector J, Liu X, Gardner EL: Electrical and chemical stimulation of the basolateral complex of the amygdala reinstates cocaine-seeking behavior in the rat. Psychopharmacology 2003;168:75–83.

166 Koob GF: Stress, corticotropin-releasing factor, and drug addiction. Ann NY Acad Sci 1999;897: 27–45.

167 Heilig M, Koob GF: A key role for corticotropin-releasing factor in alcohol dependence. Trends Neurosci 2007;30:399–406.

168 Koob GF, Zorrilla EP: Neurobiological mechanisms of addiction: focus on corticotropin-releasing factor. Curr Opin Investig Drugs 2010;11: 63–71.

169 Grimm JW, Hope BT, Wise RA, Shaham Y: Neuroadaptation: incubation of cocaine craving after withdrawal. Nature 2001;412:141–142.

170 Grimm JW, Lu L, Hayashi T, Hope BT, Su T-P, Shaham Y: Time-dependent increases in brain-derived neurotrophic factor protein levels within the mesolimbic dopamine system after withdrawal from cocaine: implications for incubation of cocaine craving. J Neurosci 2003;23:742–747.

171 Lu L, Hope BT, Dempsey J, Liu SY, Bossert JM, Shaham Y: Central amygdala ERK signaling pathway is critical to incubation of cocaine craving. Nat Neurosci 2005;8:212–219.

172 Lu L, Uejima JL, Gray SM, Bossert JM, Shaham Y: Systemic and central amygdala injections of the $mGluR_{2/3}$ agonist LY379268 attenuate the expression of incubation of cocaine craving. Biol Psychiatry 2007;61:591–598.

173 Xi Z-X, Gilbert J, Campos AC, Kline N, Ashby CR Jr, Hagan JJ, Heidbreder CA, Gardner EL: Blockade of mesolimbic dopamine D_3 receptors inhibits stress-induced reinstatement of cocaine-seeking in rats. Psychopharmacology 2004;176:57–65.

174 Hebb DO: The Organization of Behavior. A Neuropsychological Theory. New York, Wiley, 1949.

175 Chen BT, Hopf W, Bonci A: Synaptic plasticity in the mesolimbic system: therapeutic implications for substance abuse. Ann NY Acad Sci 2010;1187: 129–139.

176 Thomas MJ, Beurrier C, Bonci A, Malenka RC: Long-term depression in the nucleus accumbens: a neural correlate of behavioral sensitization to cocaine. Nat Neurosci 2001;4:1217–1223.

177 Hoffman AF, Oz M, Caulder T, Lupica CR: Functional tolerance and blockade of long-term depression at synapses in the nucleus accumbens after chronic cannabinoid Exposure. J Neurosci 2003;23:4815–4820.

178 Fourgeaud L, Mato S, Bouchet D, Hémar A, Worley PF, Manzoni OJ: A single in vivo exposure to cocaine abolishes endocannabinoid-mediated long-term depression in the nucleus accumbens. J Neurosci 2004;24:6939–6945.

179 Liu Q-S, Pu L, Poo M-M: Repeated cocaine exposure in vivo facilitates LTP induction in midbrain dopamine neurons. Nature 2005;437:1027–1031.

180 Tye KM, Stuber GD, de Ridder B, Bonci A, Janak PH: Rapid strengthening of thalamo-amygdala synapses mediates cue-reward learning. Nature 2008;453:1253–1258.

181 Rademacher DJ, Rosenkranz JA, Morshedi MM, Sullivan EM, Meredith GE: Amphetamine-associated contextual learning is accompanied by structural and functional plasticity in the basolateral amygdala. J Neurosci 2010;30:4676–4686.

182 Pu L, Bao G-B, Xu N-J, Ma L, Pei G: Hippocampal long-term potentiation is reduced by chronic opiate treatment and can be restored by re-exposure to opiates. J Neurosci 2002;22:1914–1921.

183 Thompson AM, Swant J, Gosnell BA, Wagner JJ: Modulation of long-term potentiation in the rat hippocampus following cocaine self-administration. Neuroscience 2004;127:177–185.

184 Kenney JW, Gould TJ: Modulation of hippocampus-dependent learning and synaptic plasticity by nicotine. Mol Neurobiol 2008;38:101–121.

185 Kasanetz F, Deroche-Gamonet V, Berson N, Balado E, Lafourcade M, Manzoni O, Piazza PV: Transition to addiction is associated with a persistent impairment in synaptic plasticity. Science 2010;328: 1709–1712.

186 Gardner EL: Pain management and the so-called 'risk' of addiction; in Smith H, Passik SD (eds): Pain and Chemical Dependency. London, Oxford University Press, 2008, pp 427–435.

187 Narita M, Kishimoto Y, Ise Y, Yajima Y, Misawa K, Suzuki T: Direct evidence for the involvement of the mesolimbic κ-opioid system in the morphine-induced rewarding effect under an inflammatory pain-like state. Neuropsychopharmacology 2005;30: 111–118.

188 Ozaki S, Narita M, Narita M, Ozaki M, Khotib J, Suzuki T: Role of extracellular signal-regulated kinase in the ventral tegmental area in the suppression of the morphine-induced rewarding effect in mice with sciatic nerve ligation. J Neurochem 2004; 88:1389–1397.

189 Kinshore KR, Desiraju T: Inhibition of positively rewarding behavior by the heightened aggressive state evoked either by pain-inducing stimulus or septal lesion. Indian J Physiol Pharmacol 1990;34: 125–129.

190 Vaccarino AL, Marek P, Kest B, Ben-Eliyahu S, Couret LC Jr, Kao B, Liebeskind JC: Morphine fails to produce tolerance when administered in the presence of formalin pain in rats. Brain Res 1993; 627:287–290.

191 UNAIDS (Joint United Nations Programme on HIV/AIDS): Cancer Pain Relief, with a Guide to Opioid Availability, ed 2. Geneva, World Health Organization, 1996, pp 24–37.

192 Stotts AL, Dodrill CL, Kosten TR: Opioid dependence treatment: options in pharmacotherapy. Expert Opin Pharmacother 2009;10:1727–1740.

193 Lobmaier P, Gossop M, Waal H, Bramness J: The pharmacological treatment of opioid addiction: a clinical perspective. Eur J Clin Pharmacol 2010;66: 537–545.

194 Wakhlu S: Buprenorphine: a review. J Opioid Manag 2009;5:59–64.

195 Strang J, Metrebian N, Lintzeris N, Potts L, Carnwath T, Mayet S, Williams H, Zador D, Evers R, Groshkova T, Charles V, Martin A, Forzisi L: Supervised injectable heroin or injectable methadone versus optimised oral methadone as treatment for chronic heroin addicts in England after persistent failure in orthodox treatment (RIOTT): a randomised trial. Lancet 2010;375:1885–1895.

196 Ross S, Peselow E: Pharmacotherapy of addictive disorders. Clin Neuropharmacol 2009;32:277–289.

197 O'Brien CP: Anticraving medications for relapse prevention: a possible new class of psychoactive medications. Am J Psychiatry 2005;162: 1423–1431.

198 Ray LA, Chin PF, Miotto K: Naltrexone for the treatment of alcoholism: clinical findings, mechanisms of action, and pharmacogenetics. CNS Neurol Disord Drug Targets 2010;9:13–22.

199 Altshuler HL, Phillips PA, Feinhandler DA: Alteration of ethanol self-administration by naltrexone. Life Sci 1980;26:679–688.

200 Gonzales RA, Weiss F: Suppression of ethanol-reinforced behavior by naltrexone is associated with attenuation of the ethanol-induced increase in dialysate dopamine levels in the nucleus accumbens. J Neurosci 1998;18:10663–10671.

201 Roberts AJ, McDonald JS, Heyser CJ, Kieffer BL, Matthes HWD, Koob GF, Gold LH: μ-Opioid receptor knockout mice do not self-administer alcohol. J Pharmacol Exp Ther 2000;293:1002–1008.

202 Gardner EL, Paredes W, Smith D, Zukin RS: Facilitation of brain stimulation reward by Δ^9-tetrahydrocannabinol is mediated by an endogenous opioid mechanism. Adv Biosci 1989;75:671–674.

203 Chen J, Paredes W, Li J, Smith D, Lowinson J, Gardner EL: Δ^9-Tetrahydrocannabinol produces naloxone-blockable enhancement of presynaptic basal dopamine efflux in nucleus accumbens of conscious, freely-moving rats as measured by intracerebral microdialysis. Psychopharmacology 1990;102:156–162.

204 Tanda G, Pontieri FE, di Chiara G: Cannabinoid and heroin activation of mesolimbic dopamine transmission by a common μ_1 opioid receptor mechanism. Science 1997;276:2048–2050.

205 Mason BJ, Heyser CJ: Acamprosate: a prototypic neuromodulator in the treatment of alcohol dependence. CNS Neurol Disord Drug Targets 2010;9:23–32.

206 Ameisen O: Complete and prolonged suppression of symptoms and consequences of alcohol-dependence using high-dose baclofen: a self-case report of a physician. Alcohol Alcohol 2005;40:147–150.

207 Ameisen O: The End of My Addiction. New York, Farrar, Straus and Giroux, 2008.

208 Addolorato G, Leggio L: Safety and efficacy of baclofen in the treatment of alcohol-dependent patients. Curr Pharm Des 2010;16:2113–2117.

209 Mason BJ, Heyser CJ: The neurobiology, clinical efficacy and safety of acamprosate in the treatment of alcohol dependence. Expert Opin Drug Saf 2010; 9:177–188.

210 Roberts DCS, Andrews MM, Vickers GJ: Baclofen attenuates the reinforcing effects of cocaine in rats. Neuropsychopharmacology 1996;15:417–423.

211 Roberts DCS, Andrews MM: Baclofen suppression of cocaine self-administration: demonstration using a discrete trials procedure. Psychopharmacology 1997;131:271–277.

212 Brebner K, Phelan R, Roberts DCS: Intra-VTA baclofen attenuates cocaine self-administration on a progressive ratio schedule of reinforcement. Pharmacol Biochem Behav 2000;66:857–862.

213 Brebner K, Phelan R, Roberts DCS: Effect of baclofen on cocaine self-administration in rats reinforced under fixed-ratio 1 and progressive-ratio schedules. Psychopharmacology 2000;148: 314–321.

214 Roberts DCS, Brebner K: GABA modulation of cocaine self-administration. Ann NY Acad Sci 2000; 909:145–158.

215 Cousins MS, Roberts DCS, de Wit H: $GABA_B$ receptor agonists for the treatment of drug addiction: a review of recent findings. Drug Alcohol Depend 2002;65:209–220.

216 Jorenby DE, Hays JT, Rigotti NA, Azoulay S, Watsky EJ, Williams KE, Billing CB, Gong J, Reeves KR: Efficacy of varenicline, an $\alpha_4\beta_2$ nicotinic acetylcholine receptor partial agonist, vs placebo or sustained-release bupropion for smoking cessation: a randomized controlled trial. JAMA 2006;296: 56–63.

217 Garrison GD, Dugan SE: Varenicline: a first-line treatment option for smoking cessation. Clin Ther 2009;31:463–491.

218 Spiller K, Xi ZX, Li X, Ashby CR Jr, Callahan PM, Tehim A, Gardner EL: Varenicline attenuates nicotine-enhanced brain-stimulation reward by activation of $\alpha_4\beta_2$ nicotinic receptors in rats. Neuropharmacology 2009;57:60–66.

219 Glynn DA, Cryan JF, Kent P, Flynn RA, Kennedy MP: Update on smoking cessation therapies. Adv Ther 2009;26:369–382.

220 Meyer JH, Goulding VS, Wilson AA, Hussey D, Christensen BK, Houle S: Bupropion occupancy of the dopamine transporter is low during clinical treatment. Psychopharmacology 2002;163: 102–105.

221 Semmer JE, Martin BR, Damaj MI: Bupropion is a nicotinic antagonist. J Pharmacol Exp Ther 2000; 295:321–327.

222 Froimowitz M, Wu KM, Moussa A, Haidar RM, Jurayj J, George C, Gardner EL: Slow-onset, long-duration 3-(3′,4′-dichlorophenyl)-1-indanamine monoamine reuptake blockers as potential medications to treat cocaine abuse. J Med Chem 2000;43: 4981–4992.

223 Desai RI, Kopajtic TA, Koffarnus M, Newman AH, Katz JL: Identification of a dopamine transporter ligand that blocks the stimulant effects of cocaine. J Neurosci 2005;25:1889–1893.

224 Gardner EL, Liu X, Paredes W, Giordano A, Spector J, Lepore M, Wu KM, Froimowitz M: A slow-onset, long-duration indanamine monoamine reuptake inhibitor as a potential maintenance pharmacotherapy for psychostimulant abuse: effects in laboratory rat models relating to addiction. Neuropharmacology 2006;51:993–1003.

225 Tanda G, Newman AH, Katz JL: Discovery of drugs to treat cocaine dependence: behavioral and neurochemical effects of atypical dopamine transport inhibitors. Adv Pharmacol 2009;57:253–289.

226 Peng X-Q, Xi Z-X, Li X, Spiller K, Li J, Chun L, Wu K-M, Froimowitz M, Gardner EL: Is slow-onset long-acting monoamine transport blockade to cocaine as methadone is to heroin? Implication for anti-addiction medications. Neuropsychopharmacology 2010;35:2564–2578.

227 Carlezon WA Jr, Wise RA: Rewarding actions of phencyclidine and related drugs in nucleus accumbens shell and frontal cortex. J Neurosci 1996;16: 3112–3122.

228 Kushner SA, Dewey SL, Kornetsky C: Gamma-vinyl GABA attenuates cocaine-induced lowering of brain stimulation reward thresholds. Psychopharmacology 1997;133:383–388.

229 Dewey SL, Morgan AE, Ashby CR Jr, Horan B, Kushner SA, Logan J, Volkow ND, Fowler JS, Gardner EL, Brodie JD: A novel strategy for the treatment of cocaine addiction. Synapse 1998;30:119–129.

230 Dewey SL, Brodie JD, Gerasimov M, Horan B, Gardner EL, Ashby CR Jr: A pharmacologic strategy for the treatment of nicotine addiction. Synapse 1999;31:76–86.

231 Kushner SA, Dewey SL, Kornetsky C: The irreversible γ-aminobutyric acid (GABA) transaminase inhibitor γ-vinyl-GABA blocks cocaine self-administration in rats. J Pharmacol Exp Ther 1999;290:797–802.

232 Gerasimov MR, Ashby CR Jr, Gardner EL, Mills MJ, Brodie JD, Dewey SL: Gamma-vinyl GABA inhibits methamphetamine, heroin, or ethanol-induced increases in nucleus accumbens dopamine. Synapse 1999;34:11–19.

233 Paul M, Dewey SL, Gardner EL, Brodie JD, Ashby CR Jr: Gamma-vinyl GABA (GVG) blocks expression of the conditioned place preference response to heroin in rats. Synapse 2001;41:219–220.

234 Gardner EL, Schiffer WK, Horan BA, Highfield D, Dewey SL, Brodie JD, Ashby CR Jr: Gamma-vinyl GABA, an irreversible inhibitor of GABA transaminase, alters the acquisition and expression of cocaine-induced sensitization in male rats. Synapse 2002;46:240–250.

235 Brodie JD, Figueroa E, Dewey SL: Treating cocaine addiction: from preclinical to clinical trial experience with gamma-vinyl GABA. Synapse 2003;50: 261–265.

236 Peng X-Q, Li X, Gilbert JG, Pak AC, Ashby CR Jr, Brodie JD, Dewey SL, Gardner EL, Xi Z-X: Gamma-vinyl GABA inhibits cocaine-triggered reinstatement of drug-seeking behavior in rats by a non-dopaminergic mechanism. Drug Alcohol Depend 2008;97:216–225.

237 DeMarco A, Dalal RM, Pai J, Aquilina SD, Mullapudi U, Hammel C, Kothari SK, Kahanda M, Liebling CN, Patel V, Schiffer WK, Brodie JD, Dewey SL: Racemic gamma vinyl-GABA (R,S-GVG) blocks methamphetamine-triggered reinstatement of conditioned place preference. Synapse 2009;63:87–94.

238 Brodie JD, Case BG, Figueroa E, Dewey SL, Robinson JA, Wanderling JA, Laska EM: Randomized, double-blind, placebo-controlled trial of vigabatrin for the treatment of cocaine dependence in Mexican parolees. Am J Psychiatry 2009; 166:1269–1277.

239 Gardner EL, Paredes W, Smith D, Donner A, Milling C, Cohen D, Morrison D: Facilitation of brain stimulation reward by Δ^9-tetrahydrocannabinol. Psychopharmacology 1988; 96:142–144.

240 Gardner EL, Lowinson JH: Marijuana's interaction with brain reward systems: update 1991. Pharmacol Biochem Behav 1991;40:571–580.

241 Lepore M, Vorel SR, Lowinson J, Gardner EL: Conditioned place preference induced by Δ^9-tetrahydrocannabinol: comparison with cocaine, morphine, and food reward. Life Sci 1995;56: 2073–2080.

242 de Vries TJ, Homberg JR, Binnekade R, Raasø H, Schoffelmeer ANM: Cannabinoid modulation of the reinforcing and motivational properties of heroin and heroin-associated cues in rats. Psychopharmacology 2003;168:164–169.

243 Fattore L, Spano MS, Cossu G, Deiana S, Fratta W: Cannabinoid mechanism in reinstatement of heroin-seeking after a long period of abstinence in rats. Eur J Neurosci 2003;17:1723–1726.

244 Anggadiredja K, Nakamichi M, Hiranita T, Tanaka H, Shoyama Y, Watanabe S, Yamamoto T: Endocannabinoid system modulates relapse to methamphetamine seeking: possible mediation by the arachidonic acid cascade. Neuropsychopharmacology 2004;29:1470–1478.

245 Spano MS, Fattore L, Cossu G, Deiana S, Fadda P, Fratta W: CB1 receptor agonist and heroin, but not cocaine, reinstate cannabinoid-seeking behaviour in the rat. Br J Pharmacol 2004;143:343–350.

246 Yamamoto T, Anggadiredja K, Hiranita T: New perspectives in the studies on endocannabinoid and cannabis: a role for the endocannabinoid-arachidonic acid pathway in drug reward and long-lasting relapse to drug taking. J Pharmacol Sci 2004;96:382–388.

247 Gardner EL: Endocannabinoid signaling system and brain reward: emphasis on dopamine. Pharmacol Biochem Behav 2005;81:263–284.

248 Fattore L, Spano S, Cossu G, Deiana S, Fadda P, Fratta W: Cannabinoid CB_1 antagonist SR 141716A attenuates reinstatement of heroin self-administration in heroin-abstinent rats. Neuropharmacology 2005;48:1097–1104.

249 le Foll B, Goldberg SR: Cannabinoid CB_1 receptor antagonists as promising new medications for drug dependence. J Pharmacol Exp Ther 2005;312: 875–883.

250 Economidou D, Mattioli L, Cifani C, Perfumi M, Massi M, Cuomo V, Trabace L, Ciccocioppo R: Effect of the cannabinoid CB_1 receptor antagonist SR-141716A on ethanol self-administration and ethanol-seeking behaviour in rats. Psychopharmacology 2006;183:394–403.

251 Fagerström K, Balfour DJ: Neuropharmacology and potential efficacy of new treatments for tobacco dependence. Exp Opin Investig Drugs 2006;15: 107–116.

252 Li X, Hoffman AF, Peng X-Q, Lupica CR, Gardner EL, Xi Z-X: Attenuation of basal and cocaine-enhanced locomotion and nucleus accumbens dopamine in cannabinoid CB1-receptor-knockout mice. Psychopharmacology 2009;204:1–11.

253 Uys JD, LaLumiere RT: Glutamate: the new frontier in pharmacotherapy for cocaine addiction. CNS Neurol Disord Drug Targets 2008;7:482–491.

254 Kalivas PW: The glutamate homeostasis hypothesis of addiction. Nat Rev Neurosci 2009;10:561–572.

255 Kalivas PW, Lalumiere RT, Knackstedt L, Shen H: Glutamate transmission in addiction. Neuropharmacology 2009;56(suppl 1):169–173.

256 Knackstedt LA, Kalivas PW: Glutamate and reinstatement. Curr Opin Pharmacol 2009;9:59–64.

257 Olive MF: Metabotropic glutamate receptor ligands as potential therapeutics for addiction. Curr Drug Abuse Rev 2009;2:83–98.

258 Moussawi K, Kalivas PW: Group II metabotropic glutamate receptors (mGlu2/3) in drug addiction. Eur J Pharmacol 2010;639:115–122.

259 Schmidt HD, Pierce RC: Cocaine-induced neuroadaptations in glutamate transmission: potential therapeutic targets for craving and addiction. Ann NY Acad Sci 2010;1187:35–75.

260 Wise RA, Morales M: A ventral tegmental CRF-glutamate-dopamine interaction in addiction. Brain Res 2010;1314:38–43.

261 Li X, Gardner EL, Xi Z-X: The metabotropic glutamate receptor 7 ($mGluR_7$) allosteric agonist AMN082 modulates nucleus accumbens GABA and glutamate, but not dopamine, in rats. Neuropharmacology 2008;54:542–551.

262 Li X, Li J, Gardner EL, Xi Z-X: Activation of mGluR7s inhibits cocaine-induced reinstatement of drug-seeking behavior by a nucleus accumbens glutamate-mGluR2/3 mechanism in rats. J Neurochem 2010;114:1368–1380.

263 Peng X-Q, Li J, Gardner EL, Ashby CR Jr, Thomas A, Wozniak K, Slusher BS, Xi Z-X: Oral administration of the NAALADase inhibitor GPI-5693 attenuates cocaine-induced reinstatement of drug-seeking behavior in rats. Eur J Pharmacol 2010;627: 156–161.

264 Xi Z-X, Kiyatkin M, Li X, Peng X-Q, Wiggins A, Spiller K, Li J, Gardner EL: N-acetyl-aspartatylglutamate (NAAG) attenuates cocaine-enhanced brain-stimulation reward and cocaine self-administration in rats. Neuropharmacology 2010;58:304–313.

265 Xi Z-X, Li X, Peng X-Q, Li J, Chun L, Gardner EL, Thomas AG, Slusher BS, Ashby CR Jr: Inhibition of NAALADase by 2-PMPA attenuates cocaine-induced relapse in rats: a NAAG-mGluR2/3-mediated mechanism. J Neurochem 2010;112: 564–576.

266 Valdez GR, Koob GF: Allostasis and dysregulation of corticotropin-releasing factor and neuropeptide Y systems: implications for the development of alcoholism. Pharmacol Biochem Behav 2004;79: 671–689.

267 Funk CK, O'Dell LE, Crawford EF, Koob GF: Corticotropin-releasing factor within the central nucleus of the amygdala mediates enhanced ethanol self-administration in withdrawn, ethanol-dependent rats. J Neurosci 2006;26:11324–11332.

268 Chu K, Koob GF, Cole M, Zorrilla EP, Roberts AJ: Dependence-induced increases in ethanol self-administration in mice are blocked by the CRF_1 receptor antagonist antalarmin and by CRF_1 receptor knockout. Pharmacol Biochem Behav 2007;86: 813–821.

269 Funk CK, Zorrilla EP, Lee MJ, Rice KC, Koob GF: Corticotropin-releasing factor 1 antagonists selectively reduce ethanol self-administration in ethanol-dependent rats. Biol Psychiatry 2007;61: 78–86.

270 George O, Ghozland S, Azar MR, Cottone P, Zorrilla EP, Parsons LH, O'Dell LE, Richardson HN, Koob GF: CRF-CRF_1 system activation mediates withdrawal-induced increases in nicotine self-administration in nicotine-dependent rats. Proc Natl Acad Sci USA 2007;104:17198–17203.

271 Gilpin NW, Richardson HN, Koob GF: Effects of CRF_1-receptor and opioid-receptor antagonists on dependence-induced increases in alcohol drinking by alcohol-preferring (P) rats. Alcohol Clin Exp Res 2008;32:1535–1542.

272 Ji D, Gilpin NW, Richardson HN, Rivier CL, Koob GF: Effects of naltrexone, duloxetine, and a corticotropin-releasing factor type 1 receptor antagonist on binge-like alcohol drinking in rats. Behav Pharmacol 2008;19:1–12.

273 Papaleo F, Ghozland S, Ingallinesi M, Roberts AJ, Koob GF, Contarino A: Disruption of the CRF_2 receptor pathway decreases the somatic expression of opiate withdrawal. Neuropsychopharmacology 2008;33:2878–2887.

274 Specio SE, Wee S, O'Dell LE, Boutrel B, Zorrilla EP, Koob GF: CRF_1 receptor antagonists attenuate escalated cocaine self-administration in rats. Psychopharmacology 2008;96:473–482.

275 Greenwell TN, Funk CK, Cottone P, Richardson HN, Chen SA, Rice KC, Zorrilla EP, Koob GF: Corticotropin-releasing factor-1 receptor antagonists decrease heroin self-administration in long- but not short-access rats. Addict Biol 2009;14: 130–143.

276 Koob GF: Brain stress systems in the amygdala and addiction. Brain Res 2009;1293:61–75.

277 Koob GF: The role of CRF and CRF-related peptides in the dark side of addiction. Brain Res 2010; 1314:3–14.

278 Zorrilla EP, Koob GF: Progress in corticotropin-releasing factor-1 antagonist development. Drug Discov Today 2010;5:371–383.

Dr. Eliot L. Gardner
Neuropsychopharmacology Section, Intramural Research Program
National Institute on Drug Abuse, National Institutes of Health, BRC Building, Room 05-A707
251 Bayview Boulevard, Baltimore, MD 21224 (USA)
Tel. + 1 443 740 2516, E-Mail egardner@intra.nida.nih.gov

Clark MR, Treisman GJ (eds): Chronic Pain and Addiction.
Adv Psychosom Med. Basel, Karger, 2011, vol 30, pp 61–91

Opioid Therapy in Patients with Chronic Noncancer Pain: Diagnostic and Clinical Challenges

Martin D. Cheatle · Charles P. O'Brien

Center for Studies of Addiction, Department of Psychiatry, University of Pennsylvania, Philadelphia, Pa., USA

Abstract

Chronic opioid therapy for patients with chronic noncancer pain has become controversial, given the rising prevalence of opioid abuse. The prevailing literature suggests that the rate of addiction in chronic noncancer pain patients exposed to opioid therapy is relatively low, especially in those patients without significant concomitant psychiatric disorders and personal and family history of addiction. However, the escalating rate of misuse of prescription opioids has resulted in many clinicians caring for these patients to be more judicious in prescribing opioids. Accurately diagnosing addiction in chronic pain patients receiving opioids is complex. Managing the patient with pain and co-occurring opioid abuse is equally challenging. Diagnostic issues, current guidelines for the appropriate use of opioids in the chronic pain population and risk stratification models are examined. Pharmacologic and nonpharmacologic treatment strategies for the patient with pain and opioid addiction are reviewed.   Copyright © 2011 S. Karger AG, Basel

Chronic pain has continued to be a major healthcare problem despite noteworthy advancements in diagnostics, pharmacotherapy and invasive and noninvasive interventions. The prevalence of chronic pain is staggering, with studies indicating that more than 25% of the general population experience pain lasting more than 3 months [1, 2], with an annual economic burden of more than USD 100 billion, USD 61.2 billion of which is due to lost productivity of the workforce [3]. The economic cost of opioid misuse/abuse is also noteworthy. The prevailing literature suggests that affected individuals utilize more healthcare resources and incur higher costs [4]. It has been estimated that the cost of prescription opioid abuse in 2001 was USD 8.6 billion including workplace, criminal justice and healthcare expenditures [5].

The undertreatment or mismanagement of pain can cause additional suffering to the individual afflicted with chronic pain, but can also lead to other adverse effects including delays in healing, changes in the central nervous system (neuroplasticity), depression, suicide and opioid addiction (OA) [6–9]. Chronic pain can be considered a disease rather than a syndrome, frequently associated with a concomitant mood disorder with a risk of fatality related to the significant frequency of suicidal ideation and attempts [6, 10–15]. Recent neuroimaging studies have supported this hypothesis evidenced by structural and functional changes in the brains of pain patients [16]. Despite the magnitude of the problem of chronic pain in our society, concerns about addiction and diversion have contributed to the inadequate treatment of pain, including acute episodes, end-of-life and cancer pain [17–19]. There is even greater consternation regarding opioid therapy for patients with chronic noncancer pain (CNCP).

In the 19th century, opiates and cocaine were virtually unregulated and were prescribed and used in abundance for a variety of ailments. Early in the 20th century, cocaine became associated with crime, prompting rising concern regarding the use of opium. In 1909, smoking of opium was prohibited, but not the use of opium-based 'medications'. In 1914, the Harrison Narcotics Tax Act was formulated to regulate the importation, exportation, manufacture and distribution of opium or cocaine. In 1919, the Supreme Court confirmed the Harrison Narcotics Tax Act, stipulating that doctors could not prescribe maintenance supplies of opiates to addicted individuals. Addiction was not considered a disease state, and clinicians who prescribed opiates to addicts were censored, lost their medical license or, in some cases, were incarcerated. Addiction was criminalized, leading to consequent undertreatment of legitimate pain disorders. Years of advocacy for the humane treatment of pain sufferers by grassroots and professional organizations, along with published articles supporting the efficacy and safety of opioids in the treatment of pain [20], led to the adoption of the intractable pain statutes that encouraged opioid therapy for chronic pain including noncancer pain [21].

In current practice, physicians are confronted with the responsibility of prescribing appropriate interventions to reduce or ameliorate the suffering of patients in pain while exercising due diligence by not exposing a vulnerable patient to undesirable sequelae. Many seasoned pain clinicians and organized pain societies have supported the position that the majority of individuals with chronic pain can be managed safely with opioids with minimal risk of addiction [8, 22–26]. However, there has been apprehension regarding this position of responsible opioid prescription to the chronic pain population in light of the burgeoning prevalence of prescription opioid abuse and addiction in the USA [27, 28]. The National Survey on Drug Use and Health, and the Drug Abuse Warning Network revealed that there was a large increase from 1995 to 2004 in the lifetime nonmedical use of certain pain relievers. This increase paralleled the increase in prescriptions by physicians following accepted guidelines [29–31]. This observation supports the notion that addiction trends are related to the availability of a substance. Recent SAMHSA (Substance Abuse and Mental Health Services Administration) data [32] revealed that marijuana use was only slightly higher than the nonmedical use of prescription pain relievers, both of which exceeded use rates of stimulants, sedatives, cocaine, heroine, LSD, phencyclidine and tranquilizers among persons aged 12 years and older. The nonmedical, nonheroin opioid use among 12th graders has been estimated as having increased from 3.5% in 1991 to 9.2% in 2007 [33]. A sample of 571 opioid detoxification admissions over a 5-year period revealed that the number of admissions related to controlled-release oxycodone increased from 3.8% in 2000 to 55% in 2004. Legitimate prescriptions were the primary source of the opioids, and the prescription opioid users reported higher levels of comorbid substance use disorders, pain and psychiatric symptoms [34]. Between 2004 and 2006, there was a 38% increase in emergency department visits related to nonmedical use of pharmaceuticals. Central nervous system agents increased by 32%, and in this category there was a 43% increase in opioid analgesics, the most frequent being oxycodone combinations, hydrocodone combinations and methadone [35] Likewise, opioid analgesics have become the common class of drugs associated with unintentional, fatal poisoning, excluding alcohol, tobacco, sedatives and psychotropic drugs, but more than heroin and cocaine [36]. Between 1997 and 2002, the number of deaths related to all classes of drugs increased by 27.2%, and the reported death rate related to prescription opioid analgesics increased by 96.6% [37]. In the chronic pain population, the reported prevalence of OA ranges from 3 to 40% [8, 26, 38–41], with an estimated 3–62% of chronic pain patients who receive opioid therapy displaying aberrant or problematic opioid-taking behaviors [38, 39, 42, 43]. Martell et al. [38] performed a meta-analysis of studies conducted on opioid therapy for chronic back pain. Results revealed that for back pain, opioids are prescribed to 0.14–58% of patients. OA, as defined by DSM-IV criteria, was present in 24% of this opioid-treated population. Another often cited study by Ives et al. [40] revealed the presence of substance misuse defined by inappropriate urine drug screen (UDS) results in approximately 32% of the 196 primary care patients referred over a 12-month period to a multispecialty pain clinic.

In contrast to these findings, Fishbain et al. [26] performed a structured, evidence-based review of a group of studies examining the abuse/addiction rate and aberrant drug-related behaviors (ADRB) in patients receiving opioids for CNCP. There was an overall calculated abuse/addiction rate of 3.27% but in patients preselected for no past or current history of substance use disorder, the percentage of abuse/addiction was extremely low (0.19%). The overall rate of ADRB was 11.5%, but only 0.59% in the preselected patients. UDS data revealed that 20.4% of chronic pain patients had no prescribed opioid in the specimen. Illicit drugs were discovered in 14.5% of cases. The authors concluded that only a small percentage of chronic pain patients exposed to chronic opioid therapy (COT) develop abuse or addiction.

These conflicting data on the prevalence of 'true' addiction in chronic pain patients exposed to opioid therapy are in part related to confusion regarding the terminology ('addiction', 'pseudoaddiction' and 'physical dependence') and the population sampled. For example, a pain clinic population would likely contain a greater proportion of psychiatric diagnoses than a primary care population. Additionally, some studies used questionnaires and interview protocols that may have been inadequate, and the samples were typically small and unrepresentative [44].

Opioid Therapy – Long-Term Efficacy

In a 2010 Cochrane review [45] of the efficacy and effectiveness of long-term opioid therapy for CNCP, 26 studies were reviewed with a total sample size of 4,893. Among patients receiving oral opioids, a large percentage discontinued oral treatment due to adverse effects (22.9%; 95% CI: 15.3–32.8%) or insufficient pain relief (10.3%; 95% CI: 7.6–13.9%). Most adverse effects were minor, such as nausea, constipation and headache. Evidence of OA was reported in 0.27% of cases. Many patients discontinued COT, and there was weak evidence that patients who were able to continue opioids over a long time (more than 6 months) experienced significant pain relief. It was unclear whether quality of life or functionality was affected. Iatrogenic OA was considered rare.

Several other review articles have also shown mixed or poor results for long-term effectiveness of opioid therapy in CNCP. A systematic review of opioid treatment for chronic back pain [38] included a meta-analysis of 4 studies that evaluated the efficacy of opioids compared to nonopioid or placebo treatment. This review did not find a significant advantage regarding pain reduction with opioids over nonopioid controls. Five studies that directly compared the efficacy of different opioids failed to reveal a significant reduction in pain from baseline. The authors concluded that opioids were frequently prescribed for chronic back pain and most likely were effective in the short term, while their long-term efficacy was unclear. Kalso et al. [46] reviewed 11 studies with a sample size of more than 1,000 patients, comparing oral opioids to placebo up to 8 weeks, with 6 studies providing follow-up up for 6–24 months. The mean decrease in pain intensity was at least 30% with opioids, but 80% of the patients experienced at least one adverse effect, the most common being constipation, followed by nausea and somnolence. The short-term efficacy of opioids was judged good for both neuropathic and musculoskeletal pain, but only a small proportion of the patients continued COT. There was no conclusive evidence regarding tolerance, addiction or aberrant behavior.

A large epidemiological study [47] in Denmark revealed higher healthcare utilization costs for patients prescribed opioids. Patients receiving COT had lower functionality and worse pain than those not on opioids. An expert panel [48] recently concluded that while the evidence was extremely limited, there was a consensus that COT could be an effective treatment for carefully selected and monitored patients with CNCP.

Diagnostic Challenges

A variety of adaptive and physiological changes occur when an individual is repeatedly exposed to opioids. There is also a great deal of confusion regarding the terminology of addiction versus dependence in treated patients. The hallmark of addictive drugs

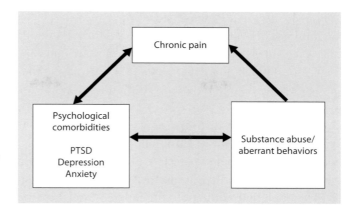

Fig. 1. Overlap of chronic pain, psychological comorbidities and substance abuse/ aberrant behavior. PTSD = Posttraumatic stress disorder.

is their ability to produce reward or pleasure. Addiction is a chronic, neurobiological disease state produced by repeated exposure to a drug that activates the brain reward system and produces loss of control over the use of the drug. Addictive drugs act through the 'reward circuits' located within the mesocorticolimbic dopamine systems that include projections into the nucleus accumbens, amygdala and prefrontal cortex. Vulnerable individuals, when repeatedly exposed to a drug with addictive qualities, develop a biological adaptation or learning that leads to compulsive use, craving and continuation despite physical or mental problems produced by the drug.

The risk of addiction consists of a confluence of factors related to the host, the environment and the agent of abuse. Host factors include genetic predisposition and comorbid psychiatric conditions. Environmental components include occupation, peer group, culture and social stability. Characteristics of the agent include availability, cost, speed of entering the brain and causing euphoria, and the efficacy of the agent as a tranquilizer [49]. There is compelling evidence that genetic factors are critically involved in the development of addiction [50]. Additional evidence demonstrates an overlap between chronic pain and psychological comorbidities, and between psycho-logical disorders and substance abuse (fig. 1) [51, 52]. Over the past few years there has been a dramatic increase in retail sales of opioids. For example, between 1997 and 2006 there was a more than 1,000% increase in retail sales of methadone, a 274% increase in hydrocodone sales and a more than 700% increase in oxycodone sales [53]. The SAMHSA 2007 report [54] revealed that in 2006, 55.7% of those individu-als who misused pain relievers acknowledged that they obtained their medication from friends and family, and that 80.7% of those individuals noted that the friend or relative had obtained the drugs from just one doctor. Only 3.9% reported obtaining the pain reliever from a drug dealer or stranger, and 0.1% obtained the drug from the Internet. Therefore, the vulnerable pain patient with genetic predisposition, con-comitant psychiatric disorders, social instability and ready access to opioids may be particularly at risk for the development of addiction or misuse of prescribed opioids.

Pain and Comorbid Psychiatric Disorders

Various psychiatric conditions coexist in the pain population, with some of the literature suggesting that pain and depression share common physiological substrates and may respond to similar treatments [55]. Estimating the true prevalence of depression in the chronic pain population is difficult in that rates vary with the population sampled (primary care vs. pain clinics) and that there is symptom overlap between depression and pain (sleep disorder, suppressed libido related to opioid therapy, withdrawal symptoms due to end-of-dose failure). Several studies suggest a robust relationship between depression and pain [56–58]. In a recent computer-assisted telephone interview with a community sample, the prevalence of chronic pain was assessed as 21.9% of the population, and approximately 35% of these patients experienced comorbid depression, which represented 7.7% of the entire sample [59]. In a sample of pain patients seeking treatment, there was a high prevalence of specific anxiety disorders identified, including panic disorder, generalized anxiety disorder, social anxiety disorders and posttraumatic stress disorder (PTSD) [60]. PTSD rates in patients seeking treatment for pain range from 10 to 50% [61–65]. Patients with psychiatric and substance use disorder (SUD) comorbidities tend to utilize opioids more chronically than patients who do not have a history of mood disorders or addiction. Braden et al. [66] examined long-term opioid use and noted rates were 3 times higher in those with a history of depression. Weisner et al. [67], utilizing health plan data from 1997 to 2005, discovered that pain patients receiving COT and with a history of substance abuse tended to receive higher doses of opioids, were more likely to be using schedule II drugs and long-acting preparations, and often were frequently using concomitant sedative hypnotics. Sullivan et al. [68] analyzed longitudinal data on 6,439 patients with similar results. Individuals with a psychiatric disorder were more likely to abuse opioids than those without a psychiatric disorder, and respondents reporting problem drug use, but not problem alcohol use, reported higher rates of prescription opioid use. Manchikanti et al. [69] evaluated 500 pain patients prescribed/maintained on opioid therapy. Anxiety was present in 64% of the chronic pain patients, depression in 59% and somatization disorder in 30%. Documented drug abuse/misuse was dramatically higher in patients with depression, and current illicit drug abuse/misuse was higher in men with somatization disorder.

Diagnostic Issues

The WHO and the American Psychiatric Association opted to use the term 'substance dependence' for what had traditionally been termed 'drug addiction'. The DSM-IV-TR [70] utilizes 7 criteria for substance dependence (addiction), with a stipulation that only 3 criteria are required to make the diagnosis (table 1). Five of these criteria are commonly observed in the nonaddicted pain patient: tolerance; physical dependence/withdrawal; used in greater amounts or longer than intended; unsuccessful attempts to cut down or discontinue use, and considerable time spent obtaining the substance or recovering from use [71]. Using these criteria in the population of patients with

Table 1. DSM-IV-TR criteria for dependence (addiction)

Tolerance
Physical dependence/withdrawal
Used in greater amounts or longer than intended
Unsuccessful attempts to cut down or discontinue
Much time spent pursuing the substance or recovering from use
Important activities reduced or given up
Continued use despite knowledge of persistent physical or psychological harm

---

3/7 required for diagnosis; 5/7 common in nonaddicted pain patients (in italics). After Heit [71].

---

chronic pain on COT is misleading. Pain patients on COT who use opioids appropriately over time will display evidence of tolerance and withdrawal symptoms if a dose is skipped or due to end-of-dose failure. These behaviors can be misinterpreted as suggesting the development of addiction [72]. Patients may also engage in ADRB suggestive of addiction to the untrained physician, but reflecting inadequate treatment of a pain disorder (pseudoaddiction). Many physicians, particularly primary care physicians, do not receive adequate training in either pain management or addiction management [73]. In addition, there is a paucity of education about addiction for medical students and residents [74]; however, there is some recent momentum to address this shortcoming in medical school curricula [75].

There was concern in the pain community regarding the potential stigmatization of legitimate chronic pain patients as having a substance dependence or addiction as defined by the WHO and DSM-IV-TR criteria. This led to a consensus panel of specialists from the American Pain Society, the American Academy of Pain Medicine and the American Society of Addiction Medicine in 2001 [76] to develop clearer definitions to avoid undertreatment of pain. Consensus recommendations for terminology included:

1 Addiction – 'Addiction is a primary, chronic, neurobiologic disease, with genetic, psychosocial, and environmental factors influencing its development and manifestations. It is characterized by behaviors that include one or more of the following: impaired control over drug use, compulsive use, continued use despite harm, and craving.' [76]. It is these four 'Cs' (adverse *consequences, control, craving* and *compulsivity*) that are hallmarks in differentiating patients legitimately using their opioids from those who are addicted. In this definition, physical dependence and tolerance are not necessary for making the diagnosis of addiction. Moreover, tolerance and physical dependence are normal responses to prescribed opioids and are not counted as a symptom of addiction. Wasan et al. [77] evaluated 613 patients taking opioid medications for CNCP. The patients were asked to judge their level of craving for their prescription medications. Results indicated that 45% of the

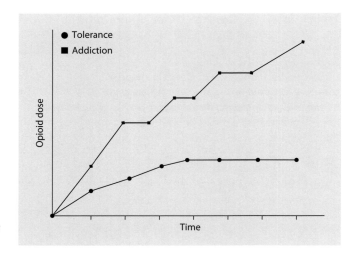

Fig. 2. Trajectory of opioid use over time comparing tolerance with addictive behavior time.

population reported some degree of opioid craving. Six-month follow-up reports revealed that those who reported craving displayed greater physician-rated aberrant drug behavior, a higher frequency of abnormal UDS and higher rates of aberrant drug use and prescription drug abuse. Craving may be a critical marker in differentiating between individuals who misuse or abuse their medication and those who have physical dependence and tolerance to COT.

2 Physical dependence – 'Physical dependence is a state of adaptation that is manifested by a drug class specific withdrawal syndrome that can be produced by abrupt cessation, rapid dose reduction, decreasing blood level of the drug, and/or administration of an antagonist' [76]. While physical dependence can clearly occur in the presence of addiction, it does not always occur. It rarely occurs with highly addictive stimulant drugs such as cocaine. However, physical dependence typically develops in patients prescribed opioids over a long time who lack other characteristics of addiction such as craving and compulsive behavior. While there has been much focus on physical dependence on drugs that stimulate the 'reward circuit', there are many classes of drugs that produce dependence without activating reward circuits (antidepressants, β-blockers, corticosteroids, etc.).

3 Tolerance – 'Tolerance is a state of adaptation in which exposure to a drug induces changes that result in a diminution of one or more of the drug's effects over time' [76]. Patients on COT frequently require increasing doses to maintain analgesia and improvement in functionality. Opioid-tolerant patients show a pattern of gradual increase in need for titration of the dosage. Patients who are addicted often display a rapid increase in dose followed by plateaus, with subsequent escalation (fig. 2). Tolerance can be present in both patients suffering from addiction and those legitimately using their medications over extended periods. Tolerance and

withdrawal symptoms are important aspects of some addictions such as alcoholism. For prescribed medications, these symptoms can be normal. Patients who are physiologically dependent on prescribed opioids can be monitored and tapered from the medication, and they do not relapse into nontherapeutic use [78].

4 Pseudoaddiction – pseudoaddiction describes patient behaviors that occur when pain is inadequately treated, including 'clock watching' and 'drug seeking'. Behaviors such as illicit drug use or deception to obtain opioids could occur in legitimate patients seeking pain relief [76]. Pseudoaddiction can be distinguished from true addiction in that the observed ADRB resolves if pain is adequately treated.

The current version of the DSM, the DSM-V (currently under development), combines OA and dependence under the heading of 'Opioid-Use Disorder'. The criteria for diagnosis (table 2) are similar to the DSM-IV criteria, except for the very important caveat that tolerance or withdrawal 'is not counted for those taking medications under medical supervision such as analgesics, antidepressants, anti-anxiety medications or beta blockers' (www.dsm5.org).

Additional Side Effects/Complications of Opioid Therapy

Common and easily managed side effects include opioid-induced constipation, which occurs in up to 90% of patients [79] but is easily managed by adjunctive therapy. Bladder dysfunction is less common, as are cardiac side effects, except for QT prolongation and torsade de pointes related to chronic methadone use, which could lead to death in a small number of cases [80–82]. Opioids can cause inhibition of humoral and cell-mediated immune responses and cytokine expression, whose mechanism involves the hypothalamic-pituitary-adrenal axis in the endocrine system [83]. Long-term effects of immune suppression are not currently known. More common and potentially disturbing complications of opioid therapy include hormonal changes. A number of studies have revealed that opioids have an effect on testosterone, gonadotrophin, estrogen, luteinizing hormone and adrenocorticotrophin. COT for either addiction or chronic pain often produced hypogonadism according to one review [84], related to central suppression of the hypothalamic secretion of gonadotrophin-releasing hormone. Symptoms included a decline in libido, infertility, depression, fatigue, anxiety and, in extreme cases, osteoporosis and compression fractures in men and women, impotence in men, and menstrual irregularities and galactorrhea in women. Patients on COT should be monitored closely and considered for alternative analgesic therapy or hormone supplementation. Many patients with chronic pain display evidence of depression, which may be reflective of opioid-induced hypogonadism and should be included in a differential diagnosis in patients with pain and suspected mood disorder. Other common complications of opioid therapy include sedation, particularly when first initiating opioid therapy or increasing the dose, most likely related to the anticholinergic effect of opioids. There are conflicting reports on the effect of opioids on sleep. Some studies have reported improved sleep quality and efficiency [85], but other studies report that opioids may cause inhibition of the

Table 2. DSM-V opioid use disorder

A maladaptive pattern of substance use leading to clinically significant impairment or distress, as manifested by 2 (or more) of the following, occurring within a 12-month period:
- Recurrent substance use resulting in a failure to fulfill major role obligations
- Recurrent substance use in situations in which it is physically hazardous
- Continued substance use despite having persistent or recurrent social or interpersonal problems
- Tolerance[1], as defined by either of the following:
  - a need for markedly increased amounts of the substance to achieve intoxication or desired effect
  - markedly diminished effect with continued use of the same amount of the substance
- Withdrawal[2], as manifested by either of the following:
  - the characteristic withdrawal syndrome for the substance (refer to Criteria A and B of the criteria set Withdrawal from the specific substances)
  - the same (or a closely related) substance is taken to relieve or avoid withdrawal symptoms
- The substance is often taken in larger amounts or over a longer period than was intended
- There is a persistent desire or unsuccessful efforts to cut down or control substance use
- A great deal of time is spent in activities necessary to obtain the substance, use the substance, or recover from its effects
- Important social, occupational or recreational activities are given up or reduced because of substance use
- The substance use is continued despite knowledge of having a persistent or recurrent physical or psychological problem that is likely to have been caused or exacerbated by the substance
- Craving or a strong desire to urge to use a specific substance

See www.dsm5.org.
[1]Tolerance is not counted for those taking medications under medical supervision, such as analgesics, antidepressants, antianxiety medications or β-blockers.
[2]Withdrawal is not counted for those taking medications under medical supervision, such as analgesics, antidepressants, antianxiety medications or β-blockers.

REM and non-REM phases of sleep [86, 87], possibly contributing to exacerbation of pain [88, 89]. COT can also cause sleep apnea [90, 91] and hypoxemia [92]. Sleep apnea may interfere with restorative sleep and place certain patients at a higher risk for respiratory depression.

Another dangerous complication of COT is overdosage. While opioids are generally safe when used appropriately, this is not true for patients who misuse opioids. In abusers, nonfatal overdoses are common [93–96]. Methadone is particularly risky when misused due to its highly variable pharmacokinetics and pharmacodynamics.

Opioid-induced hyperalgesia (OIH) is a paradoxical phenomenon seen in chronic opioid users related to a pronociceptive process resulting in an increase in pain sensitivity. Hyperalgesia is commonly seen during opioid withdrawal, but there is evidence that suggests that increased pain sensitivity can also occur during COT in the absence of withdrawal. When patients are presenting with high levels of pain on stable doses of opioids, OIH can be differentiated from tolerance by increasing the opioid dose. If there is no change in pain intensity, pain may improve with tapering and/or opioid rotation. If patients are tolerant rather than experiencing OIH, their pain will improve with dose escalation. OIH is more commonly seen in patients on long-term high doses of opioids but can occur even in low-dose opioid therapy [25, 97].

Aberrant Drug-Related Behaviors

Patients prescribed opioids may display ADRB reflective of the development of addiction or indicative of misuse for purposes of self-medication. This could involve an untreated or poorly controlled mood disorder (chemical coping), inadequate pain control (pseudoaddiction), tolerance or criminal intent (diversion). The emergence of ADRB should prompt additional assessment, heightened monitoring and the possibility of altering the treatment course depending on the underlying origin of the behaviors (addictive behavior, tolerance, pseudoaddiction, chemical coping, diversion). ADRB which are considered more predictive of abuse include: frequently losing/misplacing prescriptions for opioids; stealing or borrowing drugs; forging prescriptions; doctor shopping; co-occurring abuse of illicit drugs or alcohol; recurrent resistance to altering therapy in spite of ongoing adverse drug side effects or negative consequences of COT, and altering route of delivery such as injecting oral formulations. Less predictive behaviors include: report of unintended psychic effects; unsanctioned dose escalation (perhaps reflective of pseudoaddiction or tolerance); hoarding (possibly related to fear of not receiving opioids in the future), and aggressive complaining about the need for drugs [22, 98, 99]. One study of ADRB examined the frequency of ADRB in 904 chronic pain patients receiving opioid therapy [100]. Patients reporting 4 or more aberrant behaviors were more likely to have a current SUD and engage in illicit use. The most predictive risk factors were early refills, the feeling of intoxication, oversedating oneself and escalating the dose on one's own.

Opioid Therapy Guidelines

The American Academy of Addiction Psychiatry [101] recently outlined a number of recommendations for 'responsible practice' in prescribing opioids for chronic pain. Precautionary suggestions were rendered regarding the prescription of high-dose opioids chronically. The authors indicated that prevailing evidence failed to demonstrate long-term efficacy with regard to both pain relief and improvement in functionality, and that long-term, high-dose opioid therapy might lead to OIH as well as a risk of medical complications and deaths, particularly when opioids are used in combination with sedatives/hypnotics. The American Academy of Addiction Psychiatry recommended against high doses of opioids. Other precautionary measures included risk assessment, full history and physical examination, and particularly being cognizant of disproportionate reports of pain without objective substantiation. It was also recommended that if the patient engaged in any type of ADRB, the physician should consider detoxifying the patient from opioids.

The American Pain Society and the American Academy of Pain Medicine commissioned a systematic review of the literature on COT for CNCP and the development of evidence-based clinical guidelines [48]. Most recommendations were based on expert consensus and had only low-to-moderate quality evidence. While likewise recommending that a thorough physical examination and history be conducted along with risk stratification, they also outlined more detailed, specific strategies for patient selection, risk stratification, monitoring, informed consent and specifics of initiation and titration of opioids.

Psychotherapeutic cointerventions, both pharmacologic and nonpharmacologic, and the management of opioid-related adverse effects, opioid rotation and specific guidelines for discontinuation of therapy were detailed. They also suggested that patients may be considered for COT despite a history of drug abuse, psychiatric comorbidities or ADRB with specific caveats including increased monitoring and cotreatment by behavioral health or addiction specialists. Lastly, by consensus, it was agreed that 'high dose' in opioid therapy was defined as more than 200 mg daily of oral morphine or equivalent. It was recommended that when this threshold is met there should be more scrutiny regarding the appropriateness of therapy. Of the 25 recommendations from this panel, none were rated as supported by high-quality evidence, and only 4 could be supported by moderate-quality evidence.

Universal Precautions

Gourlay et al. [102] developed universal precautions in pain management including:
- Formulation of diagnosis with differentials
- Psychological assessment including risk of addictive disorder
- Informed consent
- Treatment agreement
- Pre- and postintervention assessment of pain level and function
- Trial of opioid therapy and/or adjunctive medication
- Routine reassessment of pain score and function
- Regular assessment of the '4 As' (*analgesia, activity, adverse* effects, *aberrant* behaviors)
- Periodic review of pain diagnosis and the development of comorbid conditions including addictive disorders
- Documentation.

Patients can be stratified into 3 different risk categories: low-risk patients (no personal or family history of SUD, no or minimal concomitant psychopathologies), who can be followed in a primary care setting; moderate-risk patients (past history of SUD, strong family history and past/current psychiatric history), who should have specialist support, and high-risk patients (actively addicted and/or unstable, major psychiatric comorbidities), who should be referred to specialty pain management centers. Gourlay and Heit [103, 104] subsequently revisited the concept of universal precautions and emphasized that this is a patient-centered model that promotes the assessment and management of treatable, concomitant disorders such as pain, drug misuse, addiction, chemical coping and other psychiatric disorders. Using this model provides an opportunity for patients to be evaluated and treated in a less stigmatizing manner and promotes the detection of complicating disorders such as addiction, allowing for the development of the most appropriate treatment intervention including the continued use of opioids.

Risk Assessment and Monitoring

Predominant risk factors of opioid therapy have included genetic predisposition, psychiatric comorbidities and personal history of substance use disorders, poor social support [105], history of preadolescent sexual abuse [106] and cigarette dependency [107]. To date there has been no evidence indicating a role of a single gene, and most would agree that the manifestation of addiction is multifactorial in nature. Psychiatric comorbidities better predict the development of ADRB. For example, Wasan et al. [108] evaluated 228 patients with chronic pain that were maintained on COT. Patients were classified as either high (55%) or low on psychiatric morbidity, and the former showed significantly higher escalations on screening tests for opioid abuse and a higher frequency of abnormal UDS results. Likewise, in an emergency room setting, Wilsey et al. [109] found that of 113 patients seeking opioid refills for chronic pain, 81% showed a tendency towards prescription opioid abuse/misuse as determined by a validated opioid misuse screener. Depression, anxiety and history of substance misuse were frequent, and panic attacks, trait anxiety and personality disorder accounted for 38% of the variance. Turk et al. [44] performed a systematic literature review of the issue of predicting opioid misuse in the chronic pain population. The strongest predictor of misuse was personal history of alcohol or illicit drug use, with moderate predictors including history of legal problems, younger age and a positive UDS result.

Risk Assessment
Risk Assessment Prescreening tools include the Screener and Opioid Assessment for Patients with Pain [110], Opioid Risk Tool [106], Diagnosis, Intractability, Risk, Efficacy score [111] and Drug Abuse Screening Test [112]. Tools used for monitoring patients already on chronic opioids include the Pain Assessment and Documentation Tool [113] and the Current Opioid Misuse Measure [114]. Available tools have

recently been reviewed [115]. Chou et al. [116] examined the validity and predictive capability of these tools and found many methodological weaknesses including the fact that the majority of the tools were validated in pain clinics, thereby reducing their generalizability to other treatment settings, and creating concern regarding their reliability in self-administered versus clinician-administered versions. These screening tools may have potential when used in conjunction with other assessment and monitoring methods including UDS, medical record audit and psychological evaluations.

Urine Drug Screening. UDS is becoming a more common method for assessing abuse potential and adherence in pain patients receiving opioid therapy. The recently published clinical guidelines [48] recommend that patients at high risk or who are engaged in ADRB (strong recommendation, low-quality evidence) and patients at low risk (weak recommendation, low-quality evidence) have periodic UDS. Up to 45% of patients receiving opioids have abnormal UDS results [39, 43, 117]. In one study [43], screening was obtained from 470 CNCP patients on opioids; 20% had an illicit drug detected, 14% had nonprescribed drugs detected, and in 10% the prescribed opioid was absent. Katz et al. [39] assessed the UDS results of 122 patients on COT, with 43% determined as problematic defined by a positive UDS result or displaying one or more aberrant behaviors. Forty-nine percent of the problematic patients were identified by UDS alone, and 32% were identified by behavioral monitoring. The purpose of employing UDS in the population of pain patients on opioids is to assess adherence to the prescribed treatment. An aberrant UDS result does neither diagnose addiction nor physical or psychological dependence. A positive UDS result alone does not predict future aberrant behaviors [39]. Absence of a prescribed opioid may be indicative of diversion behavior but may also suggest hoarding behavior as the patient may be fearful of not having future access to opioids or as the patient is potentially considering suicide.

Mental Health Screening. A great deal of recent research has been devoted to assessing suicidal behavior in patients with chronic pain [6, 10–15, 118, 119]. Smith et al. [11] assessed suicidal behavior in 153 adults with chronic pain referred to a pain center. Patients were evaluated by clinical interview and depression inventories; 19% reported current passive suicidal ideation, 13% were experiencing active thought of suicide, 5% had a plan for suicide, and 5% reported a previous suicide attempt. The most commonly reported plan for committing suicide (75%) was by drug overdose. Given the high prevalence of coexisting depression, anxiety and chronic pain, and the possibility of patients utilizing their opioids as a means of chemically coping and the potential for suicide, appropriate risk assessment should include mental health screening. Patients with legitimate pain and concomitant depression may exhibit significant symptom overlap, particularly in the somatic domain (sleep disturbance, weight and appetitive changes, change in libido and/or energy), that may lead to misdiagnosis. A consensus group evaluating the measurement of emotional functioning in chronic pain trials [120] recommended two measures of emotional functioning: the Beck Depression Inventory [121] and the Profile of Mood States [122]. Also available is the

Beck Depression Inventory-Fast Screen for Medical Patients [123], which is a valid and reliable 7-item, self-report instrument which measures the severity of depressive symptoms related to psychological, nonsomatic criteria in formulating a diagnosis of major depressive disorder. Other tools used for the screening of depression include the Beck Depression Inventory II [124], the Zung Self-Rating Depression Scale [125], Center for Epidemiologic Studies Depression Scale [126], and the Patient Health Questionnaire 9 [127] which measures 9 symptoms of depression based on DSM-IV criteria. Instruments that evaluate anxiety include the Beck Anxiety Inventory [128] and the State-Trait Anxiety Inventory [129], and instruments that evaluate both depression and anxiety are the Hospital Anxiety and Depression Scale [130] and the Patient Health Questionnaire 4 [131]. Rickels et al. [132] recently developed a 4-item screening tool for anxiety/depression for use in primary care. These 4 items had high sensitivity (78%) and specificity (95%). Brevity and ease of interpretation of screening tools are critical for adoption in a busy clinical practice. No one method has been demonstrated as significantly effective in risk assessment and stratification. Combination of UDS and the use of screening tools for mental health, functioning and risk of ADRB currently appear to be the best strategy available.

Monitoring
Effective monitoring is critical for patients receiving COT. The level of surveillance is determined by the assessment of all known risk factors. Low-risk patients who are responding to opioid therapy without experiencing adverse effects or engaging in ADRB can be monitored less frequently than those at a moderate or high risk for abusing or misusing medications or those who are experiencing high levels of depression with a risk for suicide. In these patients, the frequency of surveillance would be higher until these conditions improve or stabilize or the patients are weaned from their opioids. A reasonable monitoring protocol should include periodic UDS, a medical record audit of ADRB (emergency department admissions for pain, frequent calls to the clinic, doctor shopping, etc.) along with focused physical examination, and repeat substance use disorder/mental health screening tools.

Treatment of Patients with Chronic Pain and OA

There have been a number of studies that have examined the rate of illicit drug use in patients receiving opioid therapy for chronic pain [38–43]. One study [133] evaluated the prevalence of illicit drug use in patients in an interventional pain management setting and discovered that 16% of 250 subjects used illicit drugs, 13% using marijuana and 3% cocaine. Reisfield et al. [134] evaluated the prevailing literature on the prevalence of cannabis use and the association with ADRB in patients on COT for chronic pain. The prevalence of cannabis use ranged from 6.2 to 39% compared to 5.8% in the general United States population. Cannabis use in patients receiving COT was significantly associated with current and future ADRB, although its use as an alternative or illicit agent for pain control cannot be ruled out.

While the 'true' prevalence of OA in patients with CNCP receiving COT is unknown, prevailing evidence suggests that patients receiving COT, with no current or past history of SUD and negligible psychiatric comorbidities, have an extremely low rate of addiction [26]. Many patients will self-medicate with opioids for their anxiolytic and possible mood-stabilizing effects on depression. In fact, opioid peptides and their receptors have been postulated as candidates for possible novel antidepressant treatment [135]. Additionally, morphine used during trauma in injured military personnel may reduce the risk of developing subsequent PTSD [136]. The majority of moderate-to-high-risk patients can be managed relatively well by heightened surveillance and monitoring, and by referral to mental health practitioners and/or specialty pain clinics.

Patients with legitimate CNCP and OA are a particularly challenging population. These patients have very complex etiologies and tend to have poor outcomes from medical treatment. Jamison et al. [137] interviewed 248 patients at a methadone maintenance center; 61.3% of this population reported that they experienced chronic pain as a primary medical condition. Patients with pain reported greater health problems, more psychiatric comorbidities, a strong belief that they were undertreated for their pain, and a history of prescription and nonprescription medication use. A large percentage of these patients with pain (44%) held the belief that the prescription opioids contributed to the development of their addictive disorder. Several studies have demonstrated that poorly controlled pain in patients with SUD is associated with relapse and diminished quality of life. Larson et al. [138] evaluated 397 adult patients undergoing a detoxification program for heroin, alcohol or cocaine, and followed them for 24 months after detoxification; 16% experienced persistent pain, and 54% intermittent pain. Patients with persistent pain had increased odds of using any substance at the 24-month follow-up. These studies underscore the importance of treating both pain and substance abuse as chronic diseases. Patients with coincident chronic pain and opioid abuse have even higher rates of depression [139]. Pain patients in methadone maintenance treatment (MMT) are more likely to report depression, suicidal ideation and anxiety [140], have higher rates of psychiatric diagnoses [137] and significantly higher need for concurrent psychological treatment or psychotropic medications [141]. MMT patients with chronic pain have lower overall quality of life [140], higher levels of pain-related interference [142], and are less likely to be employed full time than other MMT patients [140]. Patients with chronic pain and OA are still often managed with opioid analgesics [143, 144]. There is little empirical data supporting an effective model of treating patients with chronic pain and OA. Most treatments of patients with pain and OA occur sequentially in separate silos at the pain clinic or the addiction treatment program. Several authors argue [145, 146] that addiction treatment without a pain management component is ineffective, and that such patients tend to leave treatment early and have higher levels of relapse.

Cheatle · O'Brien

Pharmacotherapy

Negative consequences of opioid use even for chronic pain include addiction and hyperalgesia. Tolerance and physical dependence with withdrawal can be normal. There is evidence that patients undergoing detoxification and maintaining abstinence report less pain [147]. However, there is a subgroup of patients with chronic pain and OA that benefits from access to analgesic medication.

Methadone

Methadone is a full μ-opioid agonist that blocks *N*-methyl-D-aspartate and monoamine reuptake. Methadone has long been used in the treatment of OA and also in the treatment of chronic pain. Pharmacokinetic and pharmacodynamic effects of methadone have some advantage over those of other opioid analgesics, in that methadone is long acting and development of tolerance is low, which potentially leads to lower long-term dosing. Methadone has NMDA receptor-blocking activity, and this may be the reason for its efficacy in treating neuropathic pain [148]. Methadone in the treatment of chronic pain is typically not the first-line analgesic but is used when the patient fails to respond to other opioids, there is a concern regarding escalating tolerance or signs of abuse/addiction or cost factors as methadone is inexpensive. Patients on MMT for OA who experience chronic pain typically require higher dosing. Methadone has been prescribed for CNCP with excellent results; however, this practice is not without notable risk. One report indicates deaths related to methadone increased by 390% in the 5 years from 1999 to 2004 [149]; they were directly related to increased prescription by pain clinics and also due to diversion. There are also significant risk factors in the use of methadone, including respiratory depression and QT prolongation with the possibility of torsade de pointes, causing a potentially fatal ventricular arrhythmia. Risk factors for QT prolongation and cardiac arrhythmias include patients on higher doses, drug-drug interactions or use with drugs that may also cause prolonged QT [150]. The clinical guidelines for the use of COT for CNCP [48] are very concise regarding the use of methadone. It was recommended that clinicians who prescribe methadone familiarize themselves with its unique characteristics, including a highly variable half-life requiring judicious titration to avoid adverse events such as overdosage.

Buprenorphine

Buprenorphine is a partial μ-opioid agonist and has antagonistic effects at the κ-opioid receptor. Due to its high affinity at the μ-opioid receptor, it blocks other opioids and, therefore, has been a highly effective treatment for OA and an alternative to methadone [151, 152]. Sublingual buprenorphine comes in two forms, Suboxone (buprenorphine and naloxone) and Subtex (buprenorphine) and has been approved for office-based opioid dependency treatment with the practitioner obtaining specialty training and certification. While buprenorphine has been well established as an alternative to methadone for treatment of OA, there is less data supporting its use in patients for chronic pain and OA. In one study [153], 95 consecutive patients with CNCP referred for detoxification from COT were evaluated; 8% of this population was considered to have evidence of OA. Patients were prescribed low doses of sublingual buprenorphine or buprenorphine/naloxone. Daily dosing ranged from 4 to 16 mg, with a mean dose of 8 mg in divided doses. Patients were treated over 16 months, and 86% of these patients experienced moderate-to-substantial pain relief with concurrent improvement in functionality and mood. Heit and Gourlay [152] provide recommendations for the safe and effective use of buprenorphine. It is their contention that buprenorphine, used appropriately, could be efficacious in the treatment of addiction, pain, and comorbid addiction and pain. Buprenorphine requires further research before being accepted as an alternative to other well-established medications such as methadone for both pain and addiction.

Abuse-Deterrent Opioid Formulations

New on the horizon are opioid formulations with increased abuse-resistant and abuse-deterrent qualities. These include utilization of a physical barrier to prevent chewing, dissolving for intravenous use and abuse-deterrent approaches with a combination of agonists and antagonists, typically naltrexone. Webster [154] and Katz [155] provide excellent reviews of this new technology.

Nonopioid Adjunctive Medications for Pain Control

In patients with chronic pain and OA, the prudent course of initial treatment is detoxification from the opioids and the use of adjunctive medications. Depending on the etiology of the pain complaints, a variety of medications have been shown to be effective for pain relief and improvement in functionality and quality of life. For example, in fibromyalgia, which is a very common pain syndrome, opioids are not considered to be the first line of treatment. Tricyclic antidepressants (TCA) have been found helpful initially, and newer antidepressants that have both serotonergic and norepinephrine modulation (serotonin-norepinephrine reuptake inhibitors, SNRI) have shown to be efficacious, particularly duloxetine and milnacipran [156–158]. Antiepileptic drugs have also been known to possess pain-relieving effects. Pregabalin was approved by the FDA for fibromyalgia, and the mechanism of action seems to be related to modulation of several pain pathway neurotransmitters having a role in pain processing (glutamate, substance P) [159]. In chronic low back pain, it has been established that paracetamol (acetaminophen) and nonsteroidal inflammatory drugs are first-line pharmacologic options for pain control. TCA also may have a modest effect on pain, possibly by reducing depression and improving sleep [160].

Neuropathic pain conditions respond well to the antiepileptic drugs (pregabalin and gabapentin), with evidence supporting the efficacy of duloxetine, paroxetine controlled release and milder nonopioid analgesics such as tramadol [161]. Other nonopiate options for pain management include ibuprofen, cyclooxygenase inhibitors, aspirin, capsaicin cream, topical salicylates and lidocaine patches.

General guidelines are that nociceptive, inflammatory pain responds to both opioids and cyclooxygenase inhibitors; neuropathic pain such as diabetic neuropathy, postherpetic neuralgia, sciatica and complex regional pain syndrome have been demonstrated in randomized controlled trials to respond to gabapentin, valproate, carbamazepine, lidocaine patch, pregabalin, nortriptyline and desipramine, venlafaxine, duloxetine (SNRI), opioids, γ-aminobutyric acid agonists and baclofen [162, 163]. The role of antidepressant medication may in part relate to the high prevalence of cooccurring depression in chronic pain, with the understanding that pain is a perception, and an improvement in mood will most likely lead to pain relief. There is also evidence of the analgesic properties of tricyclics and certain SNRI independent of the effect of the antidepressant on mood. TCA, SNRI and opioids are used to modulate descending inhibitory pain pathways. In a recent study by Kroenke et al. [164], a randomized control design was utilized in a primary care setting targeting patients with depression and a history of chronic pain. Interventions included 12 weeks of optimized antidepressant therapy, following an accepted algorithm, and a 6-session pain self-management program over 12 weeks. Results indicated that patients in the intervention group versus controls had a significantly greater reduction in depression and pain severity, and improvement in both pain and depression.

Psychosocial Interventions

The strict biomedical model is inadequate to effectively treat patients with chronic pain or patients with addiction, and particularly patients with both. A biopsychosocial treatment model of pain typically emphasizes cognitive behavioral therapy (CBT), a graded exercise program and rational medication management. This approach has been demonstrated to be successful in improving treatment outcomes in chronic pain patients, including return to gainful employment, reduction in pain and increase in functionality [165–167]. This same model is equally effective in treating patients with addiction and has a great potential for the population of patients suffering from both chronic pain and addiction. The biopsychosocial model of health implies that coping with illness involves a complex interaction of biological factors (exposure, injury and genetics), psychological factors (attitude, thoughts and mood) and the social context of the illness (interpersonal relationships, cultural milieu, social support, etc.).

Cognitive and Operant Behavioral Therapy
There is persuasive literature that supports the efficacy of CBT in the treatment of patients with CNCP [168]. There is also evidence that operant behavioral therapy (OBT) is effective in treating pain disorders. OBT is based on the principles of operant conditioning and on targets enhancing the activity level, reducing reinforcement of pain-related behaviors and minimizing pain-contingent medication use [169]. CBT focuses on the maladaptive thought patterns (e.g. catastrophizing) and behaviors

(e.g. kinesophobia) that occur quite frequently in patients with chronic pain and can directly affect physical and emotional functioning and the sense of suffering. The objective of CBT is to guide patients in recognizing and reconceptualizing their personal view of pain, identifying their role in the process of healing, and to encourage patients to be proactive rather than passive and competent rather than incompetent in coping with their disease and treatment regimen. CBT includes specific skill acquisition (relaxation therapy, effective communication skills, stress management principles, cognitive restructuring) followed by skill consolidation and rehearsal, emphasizing the ability to generalize these skills, maintain behavior change and avoid relapse [170].

One study evaluated the effects and possible benefits of OBT and CBT for fibromyalgia syndrome [171]. Patients with fibromyalgia can be extremely refractory to most treatment interventions. This study evaluated the effects of OBT and CBT in 125 patients. Results indicated that the patients who received OBT or CBT reported a significant reduction in pain intensity following treatment, with the CBT group reporting significant improvements in cognitive and affective variables, and the OBT group revealing statistically significant improvement in physical functioning and behavioral variables as compared to an attention placebo. Another study [172] evaluated CBT in 213 patients with back pain. Patients received group CBT, or were in a treatment-as-usual group that was given information on self-care techniques. The 5-year follow-up data revealed that the CBT group experienced significantly less pain and reported a higher level of functionality and a better sense of quality of life than the treatment-as-usual group. Economic analysis revealed that the risk of long-term disability was 3 times greater in the control group than in the CBT group, and the CBT group revealed lower loss of productivity costs than the control group. Many studies have supported the benefit of CBT for a number of different chronic pain disorders including arthritis [173], sickle cell disease [174], chronic back pain [175, 176], chronic temporomandibular disorder [177], lupus [178] and pain in breast cancer patients [179]. Insomnia is a frequent problem in patients with chronic pain, and there is also evidence that CBT has a very positive effect in improving sleep disorders in patients with chronic pain [180].

12-Step Programs

Addiction is a chronic, relapsing disease of the brain [181]. An outdated theory of addiction defined the central problem as being one of physical dependence. A more progressive view of addiction conceptualizes addiction as a problem of reward, while withdrawal plays a less important role. There is an emphasis on treatment interventions tailored to supporting lifetime abstinence [182]. Based on this paradigm, effective treatment of addiction begins with detoxification. This is followed by intensive care in a residential or inpatient program, evolving to less structured care in a partial program to intensive outpatient, and then less frequent outpatient visits. Managing addiction as a chronic illness not dissimilar to hypertension or diabetes

[183] reinforces this concept that abstinence is a primary goal. In treating patients with chronic pain and co-occurring OA, the concept is less clear regarding the efficacy of abstinence. Stress can cause relapse and poorly controlled pain can cause significant stress.

Twelve-step programs were first developed in 1935, with the original program being that of Alcoholics Anonymous (AA). The goals of these programs were to maintain sobriety and reinforce abstinence. There are data supporting the utility of the 12-step approach in combination with professional treatment. A prospective study of alcoholics [184] revealed that attending AA meetings was a significant contributor to the variance of positive clinical outcomes in the treatment of alcohol abuse. An 8-year follow-up also revealed that reduced relapse was associated with attendance at AA. A recent literature review supported the effectiveness of AA in promoting abstinence [185]. In contrast, a Cochrane review concluded that there were no experimental studies demonstrating unequivocal support for the efficacy of AA [186]. Randomized controlled trials, the gold standard, have not been possible. A variety of other programs have used the tenets of the traditions of AA and applied them to other problems, as did Narcotics Anonymous. While there is evidence that abstinence promotes better long-term outcomes in alcoholics, a case could be made regarding the use of appropriate analgesics (methadone, buprenorphine) in patients with chronic pain who are vulnerable to addiction. Twelve-step programs have their place with regard to offering a support system, mitigating frequent relapses and promoting improved quality of life. In patients with chronic pain and OA there is evidence that ongoing participation in the 12-step program, along with additional social support, lowers the risk of relapse if they receive opiates. Dunbar and Katz [105] performed a retrospective review of 20 patients with a history of CNCP and SUD treated with COT. The authors discovered that nonabusers were more likely to have a history of alcohol abuse only – or a remote history of polysubstance abuse –, were active members of AA and had a good support system. The abusers of opioids tended to have a recent polysubstance abuse history or prior history of oxycodone abuse, were not actively involved in the 12-step program and had a poor support system.

The rule of thumb is to individualize treatment based on the patient's history and levels of support. Patients who have been refractory to nonopioid treatment and are experiencing life-altering pain may require the use of opioids, which should be done judiciously and in a well-monitored and supervised environment, and they would benefit from ongoing involvement in a support system such as AA or Narcotics Anonymous.

Complementary and Alternative Medicine
Complementary and alternative medicine (CAM) approaches have become increasingly popular with patients suffering from chronic illness. Complementary medicine can be defined as nonconventional treatment that is utilized in conjunction with standard medical treatment (allopathic). Alternative medicine typically refers

to treatments that are used instead of standard medical care [187]. There has been increased interest in the efficacy of CAM interventions in the treatment of addiction and chronic pain. In fact, the National Institute of Health has established a National Center for Complementary and Alternative Medicine (NCCAM) in 1999 that 'is dedicated to exploring complementary and alternative healing practices in the context of rigorous science, training complementary and alternative medicine (CAM) researchers, and disseminating authoritative information'. In a survey of methadone maintenance treatment programs, Barry et al. [188] compared patients with chronic severe pain to patients with 'some pain', and found that both groups of patients endorsed utilizing allopathic and CAM treatments for pain reduction, with allopathic interventions mostly being over-the-counter pain medicines, and with a large proportion of patients with chronic severe pain (34%) endorsing lifetime use of acupuncture and mind/body interventions such as prayer, meditation, herbs and herbal medicine, manipulation and stretching. There is also evidence of the potential efficacy of CAM therapies for cancer-related pain, including acupuncture, support groups, hypnosis, relaxation and guided imagery as well as herbal supplements [189]. A Cochrane review [190] revealed that several herbs were more effective in reducing pain than placebo *(Harpagophytum procumbens, Salix alba, Capsicum frutescens)*. Another Cochrane review of the effectiveness of CAM for chronic low back pain [191] found that acupuncture provided short-term clinical benefit compared to a waiting list control and evidence of herbal medicines being helpful in short-term individual trials. Spinal manipulation therapy was not more clinically effective than sham treatment, passive modalities or other interventions for chronic low back pain. De Silva et al. [192] found that most CAM interventions had minimal adverse effects, but that there was insufficient evidence for any of the CAM interventions – either taken orally or taken topically – to reveal an improvement in patients with fibromyalgia. Fleming et al. [193] conducted a systematic survey of 908 primary care patients receiving opioids; 44% of the sample reported that they had utilized CAM therapies in the previous 12 months. These therapies included massage therapy (27.3%), chiropractic treatment (17.8%), acupuncture (7.6%), yoga (6.1%), herbs and supplements (6.8%) and prolotherapy (5.9%). Over 50% of the patients sampled reported that one or more of the CAM therapies were helpful. Additional rigorous research needs to be conducted to determine what subclass of patients might benefit from which type of CAM intervention.

Integrated Program for Chronic Pain and Addiction
Patients with chronic pain and cooccurring OA offer a particularly taxing class of patients to treat. A biopsychosocial model with appropriate rational pharmacotherapy targeting sleep, pain and mood disorders, along with CBT, has potential merit in this patient population. Recent guidelines on opioid therapy for CNCP [48] suggest that CNCP patients who are at high risk for OA should be treated in an integrated

fashion. There is little empirical data on the efficacy of a combined treatment program for pain and chemical dependency. Most studies have had a small sample size, but the results have been promising. Currie et al. [145] modified a pain management group program for patients with chronic pain and OA. Treatments included CBT, education, relaxation training and stress management along with exercise combined with addiction education and relapse prevention techniques. Patients who continued on pharmacotherapy were prescribed therapeutic doses of long-acting opioids administered on a fixed interval schedule. Three months following treatment, patients reported improvement in pain, craving and psychosocial severity, and an overall decrease in all classes of medications. This limited literature suggests that there is some potential benefit of treating both pain and addiction in an integrated, concurrent fashion.

Discussion

Managing complex pain patients with various physical and psychiatric comorbidities is challenging. Management of patients with pain, psychological disorders and addiction is a particularly arduous task. Addiction is a chronic relapsing disorder that involves multiple triggers and cues. Common triggers for relapse include stress, drug availability and exposure to environmental cues previously associated with drug taking. There is also evidence that stress can contribute to the development of addiction [194]. Undertreatment or nontreatment of pain in patients with chronic pain and concomitant addiction can be a potent stressor, and may consequently lead to relapse to addictive behavior. Conceptualizing both chronic pain and addiction as disease states allows for the utilization of a chronic disease management model that includes assessment, interventions and monitoring, and employs both pharmacologic and nonpharmacologic treatments (CBT, support groups, CAM, etc.). Pharmacologic interventions including appropriate psychotropic management and opioid therapy are equally vital components of a balanced approach to the management of pain disorders. Opioid therapy remains controversial, but most experienced clinicians feel comfortable in prescribing opioids to patients with chronic pain. In cases of opioid abuse, the most effective intervention for long-term success is a combined program of chemical dependency treatment and chronic pain management. Future research is needed on more sensitive measures of abuse risk in patients prescribed opioids, evaluating the efficacy and effectiveness of buprenorphine formulations for pain control in the pain patient with a history of abuse, the impact of abuse-deterrent opioid formulations on reducing opioid misuse, and the utility of a combined pain and chemical dependency treatment program. Lastly, a longitudinal, prospective study of patients with chronic pain initiating opioid therapy is needed to fully elucidate the potential risk factors for the development of addiction/aberrant behaviors in this patient population.

Acknowledgments

The authors would like to acknowledge the support from grant 5-P60-DA005186-22 from the National Institute on Drug Abuse, National Institutes of Health, for the writing of this manuscript. We would also like to thank Ms. Tracey Baum for her assistance in the preparation of this manuscript.

References

1 Portenoy RK, Ugarte C, Fuller I, Haas G: Population-based surveys of pain in the United States: differences among white, African American, and Hispanic subjects. J Pain 2004;5:317–328.

2 Pleis JR, Lucas JW, Ward BW: Summary health statistics for US adults: National Health Interview Survey, 2008. Vital Health Stat 10 2009:1–157.

3 Stewart W, Ricci J, Chee E, Morganstein D, Lipton R: Lost productive time and cost due to common pain conditions in the US workforce. JAMA 2003; 290:2443–2454.

4 White AG, Birnbaum HG, Mareva MN, Daher M, Vallow S, Schein J, Katz N: Direct costs of opioid abuse in insured population in the United States. J Manag Care Pharm 2005;11:469–479.

5 Birnbaum HG, White AG, Reynolds JL, Greenberg PE, Zhang M, Vallow S, Schein JR, Katz NP: Estimated cost of prescription opioid analgesic abuse in the Untied States in 2001: a societal perspective. Clin J Pain 2006;22:667–676.

6 Fishbain DA: The association of chronic pain and suicide. Semin Clin Neuropsychiatry 1999;4:221–227.

7 Compton P, Darakjian J, Miotto K: Screening for addiction in patients with chronic pain and 'problematic' substance use: evaluation of a pilot assessment tool. J Pain Symptom Manage 1998;16: 355–363.

8 Fishbain DA, Rosomoff HL, Rosomoff R: Drug abuse, dependence, and addiction in chronic pain patients. Clin J Pain 1992;8:77–85.

9 Mendell JR, Sahenk Z: Clinical practice: painful sensory neuropathy. N Engl J Med 2003;348: 1243–1255.

10 Fishbain DA, Goldberg M, Rosomoff RS, Rosomoff H: Completed suicide in chronic pain. Clin J Pain 1991;7:29–36.

11 Smith MT, Edwards RR, Robison RC, Dworkin RH: Suicidal ideation, plans and attempts in chronic pain patients: factors associated with increased risk. Pain 2004;111:201–208.

12 Braden JB, Sullivan MD: Suicidal thoughts and behavior among adults with self-reported pain conditions in the national comorbidity survey replication. J Pain 2008;9:1106–1115.

13 Ilgen MA, Zivin K, McCammon RJ, Valenstein M: Pain and suicidal thoughts, plans and attempts in the United States. Gen Hosp Psychiatry 2008;30: 521–527.

14 Ratcliffe GE, Enns MW, Belik SL, Sareen J: Chronic pain conditions and suicidal ideation and suicide attempts: an epidemiologic perspective. Clin J Pain 2008;24:204–210.

15 Fishbain DA, Bruns D, Disorbio JM, Lewis JE: Risk for five forms of suicidality in acute pain patients and chronic pain patients vs pain-free community controls. Pain Med 2009;10: 1095–1105.

16 Tracey I, Bushnell MC: How neuroimaging studies have challenged us to rethink: is chronic pain a disease? J Pain 2009;10:1113–1120.

17 Portenoy RK, Lesage P: Management of cancer pain. Lancet 1999;353:1695–1700.

18 Fairchild A: Under-treatment of cancer pain. Curr Opin Support Palliat Care 2010;4:11–15.

19 Deandrea S, Montanari M, Mojal AP, Apolone G: Prevalence of undertreatment of cancer pain: a review of published literature. Ann Oncol 2008;19: 1985–1991.

20 Portenoy RK, Foley KM: Chronic use of opioid analgesics in non-malignant pain: report of 38 cases. Pain 1986;25:171–186.

21 Joranson DE, Gilson AM: State intractable pain policy: current status. Aust Prosthodont Soc Bull 1997;7:7–9.

22 Portenoy RK: Opioid therapy for chronic nonmalignant pain: a review of the critical issues. J Pain Symptom Manage 1996;11:203–217.

23 American Academy of Pain Management and the American Pain Society: The use of opioids for the treatment of chronic pain: a consensus document. Glenview, American Academy of Pain Management and the American Pain Society, 1997.

24 Savage S: Opioid use in the management of chronic pain. Med Clin North Am 1999;83: 761–785.

25 Ballantyne JC, Mao J: Opioid therapy for chronic pain. N Engl J Med 2003;349:1943–1953.

Cheatle · O'Brien

26 Fishbain DA, Cole B, Lewis J, Rosomoff HL, Rosomoff RS: What percentage of chronic nonmalignant pain patients exposed to chronic opioid analgesic therapy develop abuse/addiction and/or aberrant drug-related behaviors? A structured evidence-based review. Pain Med 2008;9:444–459.

27 Johnston LD, O'Malley PM, Bachman JG, Schulenberg JE: Monitoring the Future. National Survey Results on Drug Use, 1975–2008, vol 1: Secondary School Students. NIH Publ No 09-7402. Bethesda, National Institute on Drug Abuse, 2009.

28 Johnston LD, O'Malley PM, Bachman JG, Schulenberg JE: Monitoring the Future. National Survey Results on Drug Use, 1975–2008, vol 2: College Students and Adults Ages 19–50. NIH Publ No 09-7403. Bethesda, National Institute on Drug Abuse, 2009.

29 Novak S, Nemeth WC, Lawson KA: Trends in medical use and abuse of sustained-release opioid analgesics: a revisit. Pain Med 2004;5:59–65.

30 Cicero TJ, Inciardi JA: Diversion and abuse of methadone prescribed for pain management. JAMA 2005;293:297–298.

31 Volkow ND: Prescription drugs, abuse and addiction. NIH Publ No 01-4881, rev. Bethesda, National Institute on Drug Abuse, 2005.

32 Treatment Episode Data Set (TEDS). Highlights 2007. National Admissions to Substance Abuse Treatment Services. DASIS Series: S-45. DHHS Publication No (SMA) 09-4360. Rockville, Substance Abuse and Mental Health Services Administration, Office of Applied Studies, 2009.

33 Johnston LD, O'Malley PM, Bachman CG, Schulenberg JE: Monitoring the Future. National Survey Results on Drug Abuse, 1975–2007, vol 1: Secondary School Students. NIH Publ No 08-6418a. Bethesda, National Institute on Drug Abuse, 2008.

34 Sproule B, Brands B, Li S, Catz-Biro L: Changing patterns in opioid addiction: characterizing users of oxycodone and other opioids. Can Fam Physician 2009;55:68–69, 69e1–e5.

35 Drug Abuse Warning Network, 2006. National Estimates of Drug-Related Emergency Department Visits. DAWN Series D-30. DHHS Publ No (SMA) 08-4339. Rockville, Substance Abuse and Mental Health Services Administration, Office of Applied Studies, 2008.

36 Paulozzi LJ, Budnitz DS, Xi Y: Increasing deaths from opioid analgesics in the United States. Pharmacoepidemiol Drug Saf 2006;15:618–627.

37 Paulozzi LJ: Opioid analgesic involvement in drug abuse deaths in American metropolitan areas. Am J Public Health 2006;96:1755–1757.

38 Martell BA, O'Connor PG, Kerns RD, Becker WC, Morales KH, Kosten TR, Fiellin DA: Systematic review – opioid treatment for chronic back pain: prevalence, efficacy, and association with addiction. Ann Intern Med 2007;146:116–127.

39 Katz N, Sherburne S, Beach M, Rose RJ, Vielguth J, Bradley J, Fanciullo GJ: Behavioral monitoring and urine toxicology testing in patients receiving long-term opioid therapy. Anesth Analg 2003;97:1097–1102.

40 Ives TJ, Chelminski PR, Hammett-Stabler CA, Malone RM, Perhac JS, Potisek NM, Shilliday BB, DeWalt DA, Pignone MP: Predictors of opioid misuse in patients with chronic pain: a prospective cohort study. BMC Health Serv Res 2006;6:46.

41 Reid MC, Engles-Horton LL, Weber MB, Kerns RD, Rogers EL, O'Connor PG: Use of opioid medications for chronic noncancer pain syndromes in primary care. J Gen Intern Med 2002;17:173–179.

42 Ballantyne JC, LaForge KS: Opioid dependence and addiction during opioid treatment of chronic pain. Pain 2007;129:235–255.

43 Michna E, Jamison RN, Pham LD, Ross EL, Janfaza D, Nedeljkovic SS, Narang S, Palombi D, Wasan AD: Urine toxicology screening among chronic pain patients on opioid therapy: frequency and predictability of abnormal findings. Clin J Pain 2007;23:173–179.

44 Turk DC, Swanson KS, Gatchel RJ: Predicting opioid misuse by chronic pain patients: a systematic review and literature synthesis. Clin J Pain 2008;24:497–508.

45 Noble M, Treadwell JR, Tregear SJ, Coates VH, Wiffen PJ, Akafomo C, Schoelles KM: Long-term opioid management for chronic noncancer pain. Cochrane Database Syst Rev 2010:CD006605.

46 Kalso E, Edwards JE, Moore RA, McQuay HJ: Opioids in chronic non-cancer pain: systematic review of efficacy and safety. Pain 2004;112:372–380.

47 Eriksen J, Sjøgren P, Bruera E, Ekholm O, Rasmussen NK: Critical issues in opioids in non-cancer pain: an epidemiological study. Pain 2006;125:172–179.

48 Chou R, Fanciullo GJ, Fine PG, Adler JA, Ballantyne JC, Davies P, Donovan MI, Fishbain DA, Foley KM, Fudin J, Gilson AM, Kelter A, Mauskop A, O'Connor PG, Passik SD, Pasternak GW, Portenoy RK, Rich BA, Roberts RG, Todd KH, Miaskowski C: Clinical guidelines for the use of chronic opioid therapy in chronic noncancer pain. J Pain 2009;10:113–130.

49 Vaillant GE: Natural history of addiction and pathways to recovery; in Graham AW, Schultz TK, Mayo-Smith MF, Ries RK, Wilford BB (eds): Principles of Addiction Medicine, ed 3. Chevy Chase, American Society of Addiction Medicine, 2003, pp 3–16.

50 Enoch M, Goldman D: Genetics of alcoholism and substance abuse. Psychiatr Clin North Am 1999;22: 289–299.

51 Compton WM, Thomas Y, Stinson F, Grant B: Prevalence, correlates, disability, and comorbidity of DSM-IV drug abuse and dependence in the United States: results from the National Epidemiologic Survey on Alcohol and Related Conditions. Arch Gen Psychiatry 2007;64: 566–576.

52 Swendsen J, Conway KP, Degenhardt L, Glantz M, Jin R, Merikangas KR, Sampson N, Kessler RC: Mental disorders as risk factors for substance use, abuse and dependence: results from the 10-year follow-up of the National Comorbidity Survey. Addiction 2010;105:1117–1128.

53 US Department of Justice Office of Diversion Control: Automation of reports and consolidated order system. 2006. www.deadiversion.doj.gov/arcos/.

54 Results from the 2006 National Survey on Drug Use and Health. National Findings. NSDUH Series H-32. DHHS Publ No SMA 07-4293. Rockville, Substance Abuse and Mental Health Services Administration, 2007.

55 Gallagher RM, Verma S: Managing pain and comorbid depression: a public health challenge. Semin Clin Neuropsychiatry 1999;4:203–220.

56 Kroenke K, Price RK: Symptoms in the community: prevalence, classification, and psychiatric comorbidity. Arch Intern Med 1993;153:2474–2480.

57 Bair MJ, Robinson R, Katon W, Kroenke K: Depression and pain comorbidity: a literature review. Arch Intern Med 2003;163:2433–2445.

58 Magni G, Marchetti M, Moreschi C, Merskey H, Luchini S: Chronic musculoskeletal pain and depressive symptoms in the National Health and Nutrition Examination. 1. Epidemiologic follow-up study. Pain 1993;53:163–168.

59 Miller LR, Cano A: Comorbid chronic pain and depression: who is at risk? J Pain 2009;10:619–627.

60 Asmundson GJ, Katz J: Understanding the co-occurrence of anxiety disorders and chronic pain: state-of-the-art. Depress Anxiety 2009;26:888–901.

61 Villano C, Rosenblum A, Magura S, Fong C, Cleland C, Betzler TF: Prevalence and correlates of posttraumatic stress disorder and chronic pain in psychiatric outpatients. J Rehabil Res Dev 2007;44:167–178.

62 Benedikt RA, Kolb LC: Preliminary findings on chronic pain and posttraumatic stress disorder. Am J Psychiatry 1986;143:908–910.

63 Meltzer-Brody S, Leserman J, Zolnoun D, Steege J, Green E, Teich A: Trauma and posttraumatic stress disorder in women with chronic pelvic pain. Obstet Gynecol 2007;109:902–908.

64 McFarlane AC, Atchison M, Rafalowicz E, Papay P: Physical symptoms in posttraumatic stress disorder. J Psychosom Res 1994;42:607–617.

65 Asmundson GJ, Norton G, Allerdings M, Norton P, Larson D: Post-traumatic stress disorder and work-related injury. J Anxiety Disord 1998;12: 57–69.

66 Braden JB, Sullivan MD, Ray GT, Saunders K, Merrill J, Silverberg MJ, Rutter CM, Weisner C, Banta-Green C, Campbell C, von Korff M: Trends in long-term opioid therapy for noncancer pain among persons with a history of depression. Gen Hosp Psychiatry 2009;31:564–570.

67 Weisner CM, Campbell CI, Ray GT, Saunders K, Merrill JO, Banta-Green C, Sullivan MD, Silverberg MJ, Mertens JR, Boudreau D, von Korff M: Trends in prescribed opioid therapy for non-cancer pain for individuals with prior substance use disorders. Pain 2009;145:287–293.

68 Sullivan MD, Edlund MJ, Zhang L, Unützer J, Wells KB: Association between mental health disorders, problem drug use and regular prescription opioid use. Arch Intern Med 2006;166:2087–2093.

69 Manchikanti L, Giordano J, Boswell MV, Fellows B, Manchukonda R, Pampati V: Psychological factors as predictors of opioid abuse and illicit drug use in chronic pain patients. J Opioid Manag 2007;3: 89–100.

70 American Psychiatric Association: Diagnostic and Statistical Manual of Mental Disorders, ed 4, text rev. Washington, American Psychiatric Association, 2000.

71 Heit HA: Addiction, physical dependence, and tolerance: precise definitions to help clinicians evaluate and treat chronic pain patients. J Pain Palliat Care Pharmacother 2003;17:15–29.

72 O'Brien C, Volkow N: What's in a word? Addiction versus dependence in DSM-V. Am J Psychiatry 2006;163:764–765.

73 Upshur CC, Luckmann RS, Savageau JA: Primary care provider concerns about management of chronic pain in community clinic populations. J Gen Intern Med 2006;21:652–655.

74 Fiellin DA, O'Connor PG: New federal initiatives to enhance the medical treatment of opioid dependence. Ann Intern Med 2002;137:688–692.

75 Kuehn BM: Centers to weave addiction treatment into medical education. JAMA 2007;297:1763.

76 American Pain Society: Definitions related to the use of opioids for the treatment of pain. A consensus document from the American Academy of Pain Medicine, the American Pain Society, and the American Society of Addiction Medicine. Glenview, American Academy of Pain Medicine, 2001.

77 Wasan AD, Butler SF, Budman SH, Fernandez K, Weiss RD, Greenfield SF, Jamison RN: Does report of craving opioid medication predict aberrant drug behavior among chronic pain patients? Clin J Pain 2009;25:193–198.

78 Ralphs JA, Williams AC, Richardson PH, Pither CE, Nicholas MK: Opiate reduction in chronic pain patients: a comparison of patient-controlled reduction and staff-controlled cocktail methods. Pain 1994;56:279–288.

79 Swegle JM, Logemann C: Management of common opioid-induced adverse effects. Am Fam Physician 2006;74:1347–1354.

80 Andrews CM, Krantz MJ, Wedam EF, Marcuson MJ, Capacchione JF, Haigney MC: Methadone-induced mortality in the treatment of chronic pain: role of QT prolongation. Cardiol J 2009;16: 210–217.

81 Chugh SS, Socoteanu C, Reinier K, Waltz J, Jui J, Gunson K: A community-based evaluation of sudden death associated with therapeutic levels of methadone. Am J Med 2008;121:66–71.

82 Krantz MJ, Lewkowiez L, Hays H, Woodroffe MA, Robertson AD, Mehler PS: Torsade de pointes associated with very-high-dose methadone. Ann Intern Med 2002;137:501–504.

83 Budd K: Pain management: is opioid immunosuppression a clinical problem? Biomed Pharmacother 2006;60:310–317.

84 Katz N, Mazer NA: The impact of opioids on the endocrine system. Clin J Pain 2009;25:170–175.

85 Brennan MJ, Lieberman JA: Sleep disturbances in patients with chronic pain: effectively managing opioid analgesia to improve outcomes. Curr Med Res Opin 2009;25:1045–1055.

86 Shaw IR, Lavigne G, Mayer P, Choinière M: Acute intravenous administration of morphine perturbs sleep architecture in healthy pain-free young adults: a preliminary study. Sleep 2005;28:677–682.

87 Rosenberg J: Sleep disturbances after non-cardiac surgery. Sleep Med Rev 2001;5:129–137.

88 Roehrs T, Hyde M, Blaisdell B, Greenwald M, Roth T: Sleep loss and REM sleep loss are hyperalgesic. Sleep 2006;29:145–151.

89 Baghdoyan HA: Hyperalgesia induced by REM sleep loss: a phenomenon in search of a mechanism. Sleep 2006;29:137–139.

90 Webster LR, Choi Y, Desai H, Webster L, Grant BJ: Sleep-disordered breathing and chronic opioid therapy. Pain Med 2008;9:425–432.

91 Walker JM, Farney RJ, Rhondeau SM, Boyle KM, Valentine K, Cloward TV, Shilling KC: Chronic opioid use is a risk factor for the development of central sleep apnea and ataxic breathing. J Clin Sleep Med 2007;3:455–461.

92 Mogri M, Desai H, Webster L, Grant BJ, Mador MJ: Hypoxemia in patients on chronic opiate therapy with and without sleep apnea. Sleep Breath 2009;13: 49–57.

93 Darke S, Ross J: The relationship between suicide and heroin overdose among methadone maintenance patients in Sydney, Australia. Addiction 2001; 96:1443–1453.

94 McGregor C, Darke S, Ali R, Christie P: Experience of non-fatal overdose among heroin users in Adelaide, Australia: circumstances and risk perceptions. Addiction 1998;93:701–711.

95 Rossow I, Lauritzen G: Balancing on the edge of death: suicide attempts and life-threatening overdoses among drug addicts. Addiction 1999;94: 209–219.

96 Bohnert AS, Roeder K, Ilgen MA: Unintentional overdose and suicide among substance users: a review of overlap and risk factors. Drug Alcohol Depend 2010;110:183–192.

97 Chu LF, Angst MS, Clark D: Opioid-induced hyperalgesia in humans: molecular mechanisms and clinical considerations. Clin J Pain 2008;24:479–496.

98 Portenoy RK: Opioid therapy for chronic nonmalignant pain: current status; in Fields HL, Liebeskind JC (eds): Progress in Pain Research and Management, ed 3, vol 1: Pharmacological Approaches to the Treatment of Chronic Pain. New Concepts and Critical Issues. Seattle, IASP, 1994, pp 247–287.

99 Passik S, Portenoy R, Ricketts P: Substance abuse issues in cancer patients. Part 2. Evaluation and treatment. Oncology 1998;12:729–734.

100 Fleming M, Davis J, Passik S: Reported lifetime aberrant drug-taking behaviors are predictive of current substance use and mental health problems in primary care patients. Pain Med 2008;9: 1098–1106.

101 Streltzer J, Ziegler P, Johnson B, American Academy of Addiction Psychiatry: Cautionary guidelines for the use of opioids in chronic pain. Am J Addict 2009;18:1–4.

102 Gourlay DL, Heit HA, Almahrezi A: Universal precautions in pain medicine: a rational approach to the treatment of chronic pain. Pain Med 2005;6: 107–112.

103 Gourlay D, Heit H: Universal precautions: a matter of mutual trust and responsibility. Pain Med 2006;7: 210–211.

104 Gourlay D, Heit H: Universal precautions revisited: managing the inherited pain patient. Pain Med 2009;10(suppl 2):S115–S123.

105 Dunbar S, Katz N: Chronic opioid therapy for nonmalignant pain in patients with a history of substance abuse: report of 20 cases. J Pain Symptom Manage 1996;11:163–171.

106 Webster LR, Webster RM: Predicting aberrant behaviors in opioid-treated patients: preliminary validation of the opioid risk tool. Pain Med 2005;6:432–442.

107 Friedman R, Li V, Mehrotra D: Treating pain patients at risk: evaluation of a screening tool in opioid-treated pain patients with and without addiction. Pain Med 2003;4:182–185.

108 Wasan AD, Butler SF, Budman SH, Benoit C, Fernandez K, Jamison RN: Psychiatric history and psychologic adjustment as risk factors for aberrant drug-related behavior among patients with chronic pain. Clin J Pain 2007;23:307–315.

109 Wilsey B, Fishman SM, Tsodikov A, Ogden C, Symreng I, Ernst A: Psychological comorbidities predicting prescription opioid abuse among patients in chronic pain presenting to the emergency department. Pain Med 2008;9:1107–1117.

110 Butler SF, Budman SH, Fernandez K, Jamison RN: Validation of a screener and opioid assessment measure for patients with chronic pain. Pain 2004;112:65–75.

111 Belgrade M, Schamber C, Lindgren B: The DIRE score: predicting outcomes of opioid prescribing for chronic pain. J Pain 2006;7:671–681.

112 Skinner HA: The drug abuse screening test. Addict Behav 1982;7:363–371.

113 Passik S, Kirsh KL, Whitcomb L, Portenoy RK, Katz NP, Kleinman L, Dodd SL, Schein JR: A new tool to assess and document pain outcomes in chronic pain patients receiving opioid therapy. Clin Ther 2004;26:552–561.

114 Butler S, Budman SH, Fernandez KC, Houle B, Benoit C, Katz N, Jamison RN: Development and validation of the Current Opioid Misuse Measure. Pain 2007;130:144–156.

115 Passik S, Kirsh K: Screening for opioid abuse potential. Clin Updates IASP 2008;16:1–4.

116 Chou R, Fanciullo GJ, Fine PG, Miaskowski C, Passik SD, Portenoy RK: Opioids for chronic noncancer pain: prediction and identification of aberrant drug-related behaviors. A review of the evidence for an American Pain Society and American Academy of Pain Medicine clinical practice guideline. J Pain 2009;10:131–146.

117 Fishbain DA, Cutler RB, Rosomoff HL, Rosomoff RS: Validity of self-reported drug use in chronic pain patients. Clin J Pain 1999;15:184–191.

118 Hitchcock L, Ferrell B, McCaffery M: The experience of chronic nonmalignant pain. J Pain Symptom Manage 1994;9:312–318.

119 Stenager EN, Stenager E, Jensen K: Attempted suicide, depression and physical diseases: a 1-year follow-up study. Psychother Psychosom 1994;61:65–73.

120 Dworkin R, Turk DC, Farrar JT, Haythornthwaite JA, Jensen MP, Katz NP, Kerns RD, Stucki G, Allen RR, Bellamy N, Carr DB, Chandler J, Cowan P, Dionne R, Galer BS, Hertz S, Jadad AR, Kramer LD, Manning DC, Martin S, McCormick CG, McDermott MP, McGrath P, Quessy S, Rappaport BA, Robbins W, Robinson JP, Rothman M, Royal MA, Simon L, Stauffer JW, Stein W, Tollett J, Wernicke J, Witter J, IMMPACT: Core outcome measures for chronic pain trials: IMMPACT recommendations. Pain 2005;113:9–19.

121 Beck A, Ward C, Mendelson M, Mock J, Erbaugh J: An inventory for measuring depression. Arch Gen Psychiatry 1961;4:561–571.

122 McNair D, Lorr M, Droppleman L: Profile of Mood States. San Diego, Educational and Industrial Testing Service, 1971.

123 Beck A, Steer R, Brown C: Beck Depression Inventory-Fast Screen for Medical Patients Manual. San Antonio, Psychological Corporation, 2000.

124 Beck A, Steer R, Brown C: Beck Depression Inventory, ed 2. San Antonio, Psychological Corporation, 1996.

125 Zung W: A self-rating depression scale. Arch Gen Psychiatry 1965;12:63–70.

126 Radloff L: The CES-D scale: a self-report depression scale for research in the general population. App Psychol Meas 1977;1:385–401.

127 Kroenke K, Spitzer RL, Williams JB: The PHQ-9: validity of a brief depression severity measure. J Gen Intern Med 2001;16:606–613.

128 Beck A, Epstein N, Brown G, Steer R: An inventory for measuring clinical anxiety: psychometric properties. J Consult Clin Psychol 1988;56:893–897.

129 Spielberg C, Gorsuch R, Iushene R: Manual for the State-Trait Anxiety Inventory. Palo Alto, Consulting Psychologists, 1970.

130 Bjelland L, Dahl A, Haug T, Neckelman D: The validity of the Hospital Anxiety and Depression Scale: an updated literature review. J Psychosom Res 2002;52:69–77.

131 Kroenke K, Spitzer R, Williams J, Lowe B: An ultra-brief screening scale for anxiety and depression: the PHQ-4. Psychosomatics 2009;50:613–621.

132 Rickels MR, Khalid-Khan S, Gallop R, Rickels K: Assessment of anxiety and depression in primary care: value of a four-item questionnaire. J Am Osteopath Assoc 2009;109:216–219.

133 Manchikanti L, Pampati V, Damron KS, Beyer CD, Barnhill RC: Prevalence of illicit drug use in patients without controlled substance abuse and interventional pain management. Pain Physician 2003;6:159–166.

Cheatle · O'Brien

134 Reisfield GM, Wasan AD, Jamison RN: The prevalence and significance of cannabis use in patients prescribed chronic opioid therapy: a review of the extant literature. Pain Med 2009;10:1434–1441.

135 Berrocoso E, Sánchez-Blázquez P, Garzón J, Mico JA: Opiates as antidepressants. Curr Pharm Des 2009;15:1612–1622.

136 Holbrook TL, Galameau M, Quinn K, Dougherty A: Morphine use after combat injury in Iraq and posttraumatic stress disorder. N Engl J Med 2010;362: 110–117.

137 Jamison RN, Kauffman J, Katz NP: Characteristics of methadone maintenance patients with chronic pain. J Pain Symptom Manage 2000;19:53–62.

138 Larson MJ, Paasche-Orlow M, Cheng DM, Lloyd-Travaglini C, Saitz R, Samet JH: Persistent pain is associated with substance use after detoxification: a prospective cohort analysis. Addiction 2007;102: 752–760.

139 Kouyanou K, Pither CE, Wessely S: Medication misuse, abuse and dependence in chronic pain patients. J Psychosom Res 1997;43:497–504.

140 Trafton JA, Oliva EM, Horst DA, Minkel JD, Humphreys K: Treatment needs associated with pain in substance use disorder patients: implications for concurrent treatment. Drug Alcohol Depend 2004;73:23–31.

141 Brands B, Blake J, Sproule B, Gourlay D, Busto U: Prescription opioid abuse in patients presenting for methadone maintenance treatment. Drug Alcohol Depend 2004;73:199–207.

142 Rosenblum A, Joseph H, Fong C, Kipnis S, Cleland C, Portenoy RK: Prevalence and characteristics of chronic pain among chemically dependent patients in methadone maintenance and residential treatment facilities. JAMA 2003;289:2370–2378.

143 Zacny J, Bigelow G, Compton P, Foley K, Iguchi M, Sannerud C: College on Problems of Drug Dependence taskforce on prescription opioid non-medical use and abuse: position statement. Drug Alcohol Depend 2003;69:215–232.

144 Savage SR, Kirsh KL, Passik SD: Challenges in using opioids to treat pain in persons with substance use disorders. Addict Sci Clin Pract 2008;4:4–25.

145 Currie SR, Hodgins DC, Crabtree A, Jacobi J, Armstrong S: Outcome from integrated pain management treatment for recovering substance abusers. J Pain 2003;4:91–100.

146 Finlayson RE, Maruta T, Morse RM, Martin MA: Substance dependence and chronic pain: experience with treatment and follow-up results. Pain 1986;26: 175–180.

147 Baron MJ, McDonald PW: Significant pain reduction in chronic pain patients after detoxification from high-dose opioids. J Opioid Manag 2006;2:277–282.

148 Hewitt DJ: The use of NMDA receptor antagonist in the treatment of chronic pain. Clin J Pain 2000; 16(suppl):73–79.

149 Graham NA, Merlo LJ, Goldberger BA, Gold MS: Methadone and heroin-related deaths in Florida. Am J Drug Alcohol Abuse 2008;34:347–353.

150 Modesto-Lowe V, Brooks D, Petry N: Methadone deaths: risk factors in pain and addicted populations. J Gen Intern Med 2010;25:305–309.

151 Boas RA, Villiger JW: Clinical actions of fentanyl and buprenorphine: the significance of receptor binding. Br J Anaesth 1985;57:192–196.

152 Heit H, Gourlay D: Buprenorphine: new tricks with an old molecule for pain management. Clin J Pain 2008;24:93–97.

153 Malinoff H, Barkin R, Wilson G: Sublingual buprenorphine is effective treatment of chronic pain syndrome. Am J Ther 2005;12:379–384.

154 Webster L: Update on abuse-resistant and abuse-deterrent approaches to opioid formulations. Pain Med 2009;10(suppl 2):S124–S133.

155 Katz N: Abuse-deterrent opioid formulations: are they a pipe dream? Curr Rheumatol Rep 2008;10: 11–18.

156 Arnold LM, Rosen A, Pritchett YL, D'Souza DN, Goldstein DJ, Iyengar S, Wernicke JF: A randomized, double-blind, placebo-controlled trial of duloxetine in the treatment of women with fibromyalgia with or without major depressive disorder. Pain 2005;119:5–15.

157 Mease PJ, Russell IJ, Kajdasz DK, Wiltse CG, Detke MJ, Wohlreich MM, Walker DJ, Chappell AS: Long-term safety, tolerability, and efficacy of duloxetine in the treatment of fibromyalgia. Semin Arthritis Rheum 2010;39:454–464.

158 Mease PJ, Clauw DJ, Gendreau RM, Rao SG, Kranzler J, Chen W, Palmer RH: The efficacy and safety of milnacipran for treatment of fibromyalgia: a randomized, double-blind, placebo-controlled trial. J Rheumatol 2009;36:398–409.

159 Arnold LM, Russell IJ, Diri EW, Duan WR, Young JP Jr, Sharma U, Martin SA, Barrett JA, Haig G: A 14-week, randomized, double-blinded, placebo-controlled monotherapy trial of pregabalin in patients with fibromyalgia. J Pain 2008;9:792–805.

160 Chou R: Pharmacological management of low back pain. Drugs 2010;70:385–402.

161 Namaka M, Leong C, Grossbern TA, Klowak M, Turcotte D, Festahani F, Gomori A, Intratera H: A treatment algorithm for neuropathic pain: an update. Consult Pharm 2009;24:885–902.

162 Woolf CJ, Mannion RJ: Neuropathic pain: etiology, symptoms, mechanisms and management. Lancet 1999;353:1959–1964.

163 Sindrup SH, Jensen TS: Efficacy of pharmacologic treatments of neuropathic pain: an update and effect related to mechanisms of drug action. Pain 1999;83: 389–400.

164 Kroenke K, Bair MJ, Damush TM, Wu J, Hoke S, Sutherland J, Tu W: Optimized antidepressant therapy and pain self-management in primary care patients with depression and musculoskeletal pain: a randomized controlled trial. JAMA 2009;301: 2099–2110.

165 Gallagher RM: Pain medicine and primary care: a community solution to pain as a public health problem. Med Clin North Am 1999;83:555–583.

166 McCracken LM, Turk DC: Behavioral and cognitive-behavioral treatment for chronic pain: outcomes, predictors of outcome, and treatment process. Spine (Phila Pa 1976) 2002;27:2564–2573.

167 Gallagher RM: Biopsychosocial pain medicine and mind-brain-body science. Phys Med Rehabil Clin N Am 2004;15:855–882.

168 Morley S, Eccleston C, Williams A: Systematic review and meta-analysis of randomized controlled trials of cognitive behavior therapy and behavior therapy for chronic pain in adults, excluding headache. Pain 1999;80:1–13.

169 Fordyce WE: Behavioral Methods in Chronic Pain and Illness. St Louis, Mosby, 1976.

170 Turk DC, Flor H: The cognitive-behavioral approach to pain management; in McMahon SB, Koltzenburg M (eds): Wall and Melzack's Textbook of Pain. Philadelphia, Elsevier Churchill Livingston, 2006, pp 339–348.

171 Thieme K, Flor H, Turk D: Psychological pain treatment in fibromyalgia syndrome: efficacy of operant behavioural and cognitive behavioural treatments. Arthritis Res Ther 2006;8:R121.

172 Linton SJ, Nordin E: A 5-year follow-up evaluation of the health and economic consequences of an early cognitive behavioral intervention for back pain: a randomized, controlled trial. Spine (Phila Pa 1976) 2006;31:853–858.

173 Keefe FJ, Caldwell DS: Cognitive behavioral control of arthritis pain. Med Clin North Am 1997;81: 277–290.

174 Chen E, Cole SW, Kato PM: A review of empirically supported psychosocial interventions for pain and adherence outcomes in sickle cell disease. J Pediatr Psychol 2004;29:1997–2009.

175 Lamb S, Hansen Z, Lall R, Castelnuovo E, Withers EJ, Nichols V, Potter R, Underwood MR, Back Skills Training Trial Investigators: Group cognitive behavioural treatment for low-back pain in primary care: a randomised controlled trial and cost-effectiveness analysis. Lancet 2010;375:916–923.

176 Glombiewski JA, Hartwich-Tersek J, Rief W: Two psychological interventions are effective in severely disabled, chronic back pain patients: a randomized controlled trial. Int J Behav Med 2010;17:97–107.

177 Turner JA, Manci L, Aaron LA: Short- and long-term efficacy of brief cognitive-behavioral therapy for patients with chronic temporomandibular disorder pain: a randomized, controlled trial. Pain 2006; 121:181–194.

178 Greco CM, Rudy TE, Manzi S: Effects of a stress-reduction program on psychological function, pain, and physical function of systemic lupus erythematosus patients: a randomized controlled trial. Arthritis Rheum 2004;51:625–634.

179 Tatrow K, Montgomery GH: Cognitive behavioral therapy techniques for distress and pain in breast cancer patients: a meta-analysis. J Behav Med 2006; 29:17–27.

180 Jungquist CR, O'Brien C, Matteson-Rusby S, Smith MT, Pigeon WR, Zia Y, Lu N, Perlis ML: The efficacy of cognitive-behavioral therapy for insomnia in patients with chronic pain. Sleep Med 2010;11: 302–309.

181 Leshner AL: Addiction is a brain disease, and it matters. Science 1997;278:45–47.

182 DuPont RL: Addiction: a new paradigm. Bull Menninger Clin 1998;62:231–242.

183 O'Brien CP, McLellan AT: Myths about the treatment of addiction. Lancet 1996;347:237–240.

184 Vaillant GE, Clark W, Cyrus C, Milofsky ES, Kopp J, Wulsin VW, Mogielnicki NP: Prospective study of alcoholism treatment: eight-year follow-up. Am J Med 1983;75:455–463.

185 Kaskutas LA: Alcoholics Anonymous effectiveness: faith meets science. J Addict Dis 2009;28:145–157.

186 Ferri M, Amato L, Davoli M: Alcoholics Anonymous and other 12-step programmes for alcohol dependence. Cochrane Database Syst Rev 2006;3: CD005032.

187 Kim Y, Lichtenstein G, Waalen J: Distinguishing complementary medicine from alternative medicine. Arch Intern Med 2002;162:943.

188 Barry D, Beitel M, Cutter C, Garnet B, Joshi D, Schottenfeld RS, Rounsaville BJ: Allopathic, complementary, and alternative medical treatment utilization for pain among methadone-maintained patients. Am J Addict 2009;18:379–385.

189 Bardia A, Barton D, Prokop LJ, Bauer BA, Moynihan TJ: Efficacy of complementary and alternative medicine therapies in relieving cancer pain: a systematic review. J Clin Oncol 2006;24:5457–5464.

190 Gagnier JJ, van Tulder M, Berman B, Bombardier C: Herbal medicine for low back pain: a Cochrane Review. Spine (Phila Pa 1976) 2007;32:82–92.

191 Rubinstein SM, van Middelkoop M, Kuijpers T, Ostelo R, Verhagen AP, de Boer MR, Koes BW, van Tulder MW: A systematic review on the effectiveness of complementary and alternative medicine for chronic non-specific low-back pain. Eur Spine J 2010;19:1213–1228.

192 De Silva V, El-Metwally A, Ernst E, Lewith G, Macfarlane GJ: Arthritis Research Campaign Working Group on Complementary and Alternative Medicines: Evidence for the efficacy of complementary and alternative medicines in the management of fibromyalgia: a systematic review. Rheumatology (Oxford) 2010;49:1063–1068.

193 Fleming S, Rabago D, Mundt M, Fleming M: CAM therapies among primary care patients using opioid therapy for chronic pain. BMC Complement Altern Med 2007;7:15.

194 Koob GF, le Moal M: Drug addiction, dysregulation of reward, and allostasis. Neuropsychopharmacology 2001;24:97–129.

Martin D. Cheatle, PhD
Center for Studies of Addiction, University of Pennsylvania
3535 Market Street, 4th floor
Philadelphia, PA 19104 (USA)
Tel. +1 215 746 7365, E-Mail martin.cheatle@uphs.upenn.edu

Clark MR, Treisman GJ (eds): Chronic Pain and Addiction.
Adv Psychosom Med. Basel, Karger, 2011, vol 30, pp 92–112

Optimizing Treatment with Opioids and Beyond

Michael R. Clark[a,c] · Glenn J. Treisman[a–d]

Departments of [a]Psychiatry and Behavioral Sciences and [b]Medicine, The Johns Hopkins University School of Medicine, and [c]Chronic Pain Treatment Program and [d]AIDS Psychiatry Service, The Johns Hopkins Medical Institutions, Baltimore, Md., USA

Abstract

Patients with both chronic pain and substance use disorders offer special challenges and opportunities. They represent a large number of patients with significant costs to themselves and society that translate into poor outcome. The challenges in defining addiction in patients with chronic pain, particularly in those treated with chronic opioid therapy, have distracted the healthcare community from designing effective treatment programs. Traditional treatment programs for chronic pain disorders or substance use disorders are incapable of addressing the issues of the patients' 'other' problem. Treatment devolves to prescribing opioid medications with the belief that both disorders will be treated at least in part, which is deemed better than receiving no treatment at all. Patients are actually concerned about the risks of this type of treatment, and even if it did offer significant benefits, physicians demonstrate a lack of knowledge and skill in administering opioids to these patients. The inadequate treatment of either chronic pain or addiction interferes with the treatment of the other condition and necessitates the design of new treatment paradigms. A new approach to patients with both chronic pain and addiction should start with an evaluation and formulation of these patients to determine the different domains that contribute to their disability (diseases, dimensions, behaviors, life stories). A comprehensive formulation provides the appropriate platform for the implementation of an integrated program of therapy for both conditions that can be intensified to provide more, rather than less, care for the patient that does not meet the goals of functional rehabilitation.

Is Chronic Pain a Problem for Opioid-Dependent Patients?

Chronic pain spares no group of individuals. The prevalence of substance use disorders in patients with chronic pain is clearly higher than in the general population [1]. Conversely, the lack of a standard definition of chronic pain has contributed to uncertainty regarding its exact prevalence in individuals with opioid dependence. Requiring pain of at least 6 months' duration and the pain to be of moderate or greater intensity or significantly interfering with daily activities, Rosenblum et al. [2] showed that 37% of patients in methadone treatment programs met criteria for severe chronic pain. A more recent study employed a less conservative definition of chronic pain (requiring 6 months' duration, but eliminating the intensity and interference criteria) and reported a prevalence of 55% [3]. Although rates vary, even the lower end of the range is higher than most general population estimates [4–6].

The presence of chronic pain in drug-dependent patients is not surprising. More important, it is cause for substantial concern. In general, chronic pain is associated with poor psychosocial functioning and quality of life, poor workforce attendance and productivity, increased rates of psychiatric disorders, reduced financial well-being, poor self-rated health and increased healthcare utilization [7–9]. All of these debilitating features are similarly present and probably more severe in opioid-dependent patients with chronic pain. Determining which aspects of chronic pain are most predictive of continued drug abuse as well as the comorbid psychiatric disorders and physical impairments in drug-dependent populations has been hindered by the lack of a comprehensive and multidimensional framework for the conceptualization of chronic pain [10–12].

Can Chronic Pain Be Evaluated in Opioid-Dependent Patients?

The obvious risk of patients misusing or abusing analgesic medications in the context of their opioid dependence is justifiably balanced against the substantial consequences of undertreating chronic pain. In patients with opioid dependence, regardless of whether they are receiving methadone maintenance therapy or not, the treatment of pain is disproportionately neglected [13, 14]. Unfortunately, the undertreatment of chronic pain does not limit illicit drug use and the overall severity of a drug dependence disorder, but increases it [15–18]. However, the clinical success of substance abuse treatment still relies on detecting and evaluating the misuse of prescribed opioids, which remains a challenge [19–22].

The diagnosis of drug dependence (i.e. addiction) in patients who are receiving opioids for pain management is not as difficult as many would profess. Regardless of whether the patient has chronic pain or is being prescribed treatment with opioids, a substance use disorder still manifests itself in the same symptoms: (1) loss of control over drug use, (2) compulsive drug use, and (3) continued drug use despite harm including deteriorations in function [23, 24]. While aberrant medication-taking behaviors are common in patients with chronic pain, ongoing assessment of their functioning is needed [25, 26]. If their function is stable and their actions productive, then the problems are likely being addressed, and the treatment is probably safe and effective. If their function is deteriorating, then the cause (e.g. addiction, cognitive impairment, psychiatric disorder, diversion, worsening pain, medical problems) must be uncovered so that specific modifications to the treatment plan can be implemented. This pragmatic approach to patient care in real time helps resolve continuing ethical debates over the application of well-accepted concepts of beneficence, nonmalfeasance, therapeutic dependence, pseudoaddiction and subtle withdrawal phenomena [27–29]. The question is not whether patients with substance use disorder and chronic pain should ever be treated with opioids, but how the medication should be used when the need arises.

The Relationship between Substance Use Disorders and Chronic Pain Conditions

Efforts to encourage the identification and treatment of pain by physicians in conjunction with the marketing of new formulations of opioid analgesics for the treatment of chronic nonmalignant pain conditions have likely contributed to increased rates of opioid abuse [30, 31]. From 1997 to 2002, the medical use of commonly prescribed opioids markedly increased: morphine by 73%, hydromorphone by 96%, fentanyl by 226%, and oxycodone by 403% [32]. Likewise, the Researched Abuse, Diversion and Addiction-Related Surveillance system has reported that the abuse of prescription opioids has become widely prevalent [33, 34]. Beginning in the late 1990s, a more than 2-fold increase in lifetime abuse, and a nearly 3-fold increase in past-month abuse of prescription opioids occurred in the USA (https://nsduhweb.rti.org/). Hydrocodone has become the most widely prescribed opioid with the highest rate of nonmedical use in the general population [35, 36]. The rates of nonmedical use for methadone were highest in clinical samples, where increases in methadone diversion and abuse primarily occurred with the tablet form (i.e. likely to be prescriptions for pain management rather than take-home doses from opioid treatment programs) [37].

Patients are at the highest risk for developing new drug use problems and disorders in the first few years after the onset of their chronic pain [38]. The risk is greatest among those with a history of drug use disorder or psychiatric comorbidity [39–42]. Once an opioid dependence disorder is established, patients with chronic pain exhibit higher rates of drug use than those without chronic pain [2, 3, 18, 43]. For example, chronic pain patients receiving methadone for opioid dependence were found to have higher rates of illicit drug use (opioids, benzodiazepines, cannabis) than patients without chronic pain. A more recent study examined the hypothesis that persistent pain increases the risk of relapse into substance use after a successful program of detoxification. In a 24-month follow-up study of 397 adults with heroin, alcohol or cocaine abuse, 70% reported intermittent or persistent pain, both of which were associated with increased use of any illicit substance (odds ratio = 4.2), particularly opioids (odds ratio = 5.4) [44].

Rates of aberrant medication-taking behaviors in patients with chronic pain range up to approximately 50% of those prescribed opioids [25, 45]. Despite the development of numerous self-report questionnaires, the best overall predictor of a patient engaging in aberrant drug-taking behavior is a standardized interview. These results reinforce the rationale that a comprehensive evaluation by an expert clinician is more likely to produce the best formulation of the case than evaluation by any psychometric instrument [46]. Remember, not all patients with a history of substance abuse relapse into addiction after the prescription of opioids for legitimate chronic pain conditions [47]. Future research should seek to understand the types of patients for whom prediction is inaccurate, as well as to prospectively study what happens to individuals with a history of substance abuse with chronic pain when they are prescribed opioid therapy.

What, if Any, Relationship Exists between Prescription Opioid Abuse and Chronic Pain?

Little is known about the characteristics of people who abuse prescription opioids [23, 48]. There is no difficulty assuming that pain motivates people to use licit and illicit drugs [49, 50]. For example, 45% of patients in methadone maintenance treatment believed that opioids legitimately prescribed for their pain led to their addiction [43]. In another study, 31% of patients receiving inpatient treatment for an addiction to controlled-release oxycodone reported the medication was initially obtained from a physician for a medical indication such as pain [51].

Patients in methadone maintenance treatment and dependent on prescription opioids were significantly more likely to have had a history of, or ongoing problems with, pain than patients who were dependent on heroin [10]. Of note, 24% had only used prescription opioids (i.e. did not use heroin), and the majority (86%) reported that pain was the reason they had first begun taking opioids. Another 24% of the overall sample had used prescription opioids initially, but subsequently switched over to abusing heroin. Again, the majority (62%) reported the primary reason for having started to use opioids was pain. Interestingly, this study also suggested that the patients with prescription opioid abuse were more likely to remain in substance abuse of treatment than those with heroin abuse.

Do Opioids 'Treat' Chronic Pain?

The efficacy of opioids in the treatment of chronic nonmalignant pain has been documented [52–54]. Similarly, quality of life has been reported to improve in patients with chronic pain receiving opioid therapy [55]. However, long-term opioid therapy remains a controversial practice and may be complicated by a number of adverse outcomes [56–58]. Other systematic reviews of chronic opioid therapy have failed to solidify support for this practice, citing lack of efficacy, limitations in design and sample size, and inadequate follow-up [56, 59]. Currently, over 3% of the adult population receives this therapy [60]. Because opioids have no ceiling dose due to multiple factors such as a lack of overt toxicity and tolerance to many adverse events, the titration of opioid doses is empirical. Recommendations are based on the clinical assessment of patient-reported pain relief and adverse events, coupled with imprecise estimates of functional capacity and detection of aberrant drug-taking behaviors, which are difficult to document. As a result, many patients reach extraordinary amounts of opioids with little objective benefits.

What Do Patients Believe about Their Medication Use?

Patients express concerns about prescribed opioids causing addiction [61–63]. McCracken et al. [64] studied the concerns of patients with chronic pain about medications, and the patterns of nonadherence to or misuse of prescribed medications were characterized. Overusing their medication was associated with patients having concerns about addiction, tolerance, withdrawal, excessive scrutiny of medication use by others, and a greater self-perceived need for medication. In a similar study, patients with chronic pain and a history of substance abuse were more likely to believe that narcotics were more effective medications for pain, that narcotics would improve their mood, that they would be able to function better with free access to narcotics, and that they needed higher amounts of narcotics to experience pain relief than other patients [65]. These patients achieved an about 50% pain relief and were prescribed similar doses of narcotics compared to those without a history of substance abuse. However, they were significantly more likely to misuse their prescribed medications if they believed that they required higher doses of narcotics than others and that their pain control would improve if they had control over their supply of narcotics. These findings highlight the complexity of managing patients with both chronic pain and substance use disorders. Although patients with a history of substance abuse experienced a significant reduction in pain with treatment, their misuse of medications could still be a manifestation of their chronic pain or substance abuse disorder and not simply a relapse into active addiction. A qualitative study of patients with chronic pain in methadone maintenance characterized the themes of importance to patients: an inability to obtain adequate pain treatment, having difficulty fulfilling responsibilities due to pain, and holding beliefs that methadone was causing pain. Patients often feared that other opioids taken for pain would worsen their addiction or even create a new addiction [66].

However, patients are more likely to have concerns that lie outside the spectrum of aberrant drug-taking behaviors, abuse and addiction. A recent study of over 1,100 patients receiving long-term opioid therapy for chronic noncancer pain found high rates of depression, pain-related interference with daily activities, and concerns about control over opioid use independent of poor pain control and opioid misuse/addiction [67]. In their evaluation of patients, these concerns should lead physicians beyond the obvious and immediate possibility of addiction to the larger domains of treatment efficacy, quality of life, psychosocial functioning in activities of daily living, and comorbid psychiatric disorders. A recent Cochrane Database review of long-term opioid management for chronic noncancer pain found only weak evidence that patients who are able to continue this treatment actually achieve clinically significant pain relief [68]. More important, many patients discontinue oral opioids because of adverse events (33%) or insufficient pain relief. Patients express these concerns about long-term opioid use to their physician. As a result, a recent panel of experts recommended that clinical trials of chronic pain treatment should include an assessment of overall improvement to understand the patient's definition of a successful outcome [69].

Do Physicians Lack the Fund of Knowledge for Prescribing Opioids?

Formal assessments of physician knowledge of, and attitudes to, opioid therapy for chronic pain demonstrate deficits in many domains: understanding the pharmacology of opioids, their efficacy in treating different types of pain, and the regulations that oversee their use [70]. A recent survey of physician knowledge regarding opioid analgesics found multiple misconceptions about prescribing this class of medications [71]. These concerns ranged from excessive fear of investigation, over believing certain practices were unlawful and/or unethical, to not knowing the criteria for the diagnosis of addiction. As a result, physicians admitted to limiting their care of patients with chronic pain that received opioids. For example, doses of opioids were lowered, refills were restricted, and non-Schedule II medications were preferred. The consequences for patients were very likely inadequate pain management while at the same time not being very likely to limit the perceived harms associated with long-term opioid therapy.

Physicians commonly prescribe opioids, but their expertise is undermined by their own ignorance, lack of experience and biases. Physicians worry that opioids prescribed for even a legitimate chronic pain syndrome could lead to illicit use and create a 'iatrogenic' addiction despite a lack of evidence quantifying this particular risk [72, 73]. Physician practice is influenced by state medical boards and other regulatory agencies [74]. The 2005 Pain in Europe Survey demonstrated significant differences across countries in opioid prescription practices for the treatment of chronic noncancer pain [75, 76]. Multiple factors were likely to have contributed to these country-specific patterns, including regulations restricting opioid availability, cultural beliefs, patient acceptance and medical-ethical influences on prescription. Consequences of prescribing opioids may include legal prosecution for both civil and criminal charges, further inhibiting physicians' willingness to prescribe opioids [77]. Patients presumed to be addicted to opioids are often described by practitioners as being manipulative, drug seeking and noncompliant [78]. Even to patients with chronic pain who have only a history of substance abuse, physicians are reluctant to prescribe opioids, and they distrust the patients' motives for requesting opioids and doubt whether they suffer genuine pain [79].

Before physicians can adequately evaluate a patient, they should possess a fund of knowledge of the principles of pain management on which to build their approach for the successful treatment of chronic pain with long-term opioids. A recent consensus report of interdisciplinary experts concluded that despite increasing use of opioids for chronic pain treatment, significant limitations exist with respect to evidence of effectiveness, outcome assessment and adverse drug events [80]. These limitations in evidence undermine the rationale of individual physician practices and expert experience. Educational programs can positively affect physicians' knowledge, attitudes and beliefs about pain management, leading to more coherent strategies for optimizing benefit and minimizing the risk of different therapies [81, 82]. Any approach to prescribing opioids for chronic pain should include a risk assessment that considers a spectrum of behaviors more likely to be indicators of addiction [83].

What Is the Effect of Chronic Pain on Response to Drug Abuse Treatment?

Chronic pain negatively affects the course and outcome of numerous medical and psychiatric conditions [84–86]. Chronic pain has the same effect on opioid-dependent patients receiving outpatient drug abuse treatment with methadone and counseling. Chronic pain could negatively interfere with a patient's response to drug abuse treatment in any of the following ways: (1) chronic pain might increase illicit drug-seeking motivation and drug-taking behavior with the goal of reducing pain symptoms; (2) chronic pain could increase the motivation to use illicit drugs that produce euphoria to improve subjective well-being and quality of life; (3) chronic pain symptoms and impairments could be associated with other psychiatric disorders that respond poorly to drug abuse treatment, and (4) chronic pain is often associated with disability that reduces psychosocial activity and subsequently hinders seeking or sustaining employment or attending drug abuse treatment sessions, which reduces drug abuse treatment response [18, 50, 87–93].

The prescription guidelines for long-term opioid therapy focus on principles of effective and safe use of these medications [94, 95]. The approach attempts to balance the potential benefits and risks of opioids. The basic tenets include: performing a comprehensive initial evaluation; establishing a diagnosis and the medical necessity for opioids based on a lack of acceptable response to other therapies; assessing the risk-benefit ratio; outlining treatment goals; obtaining informed consent and agreement; initiating a dose adjustment phase, and if continued, implementing a stable phase of ongoing assessment to document outcome and adherence monitoring to minimize the risk of aberrant medication-taking behaviors. Scimeca et al. [14] reviewed the principles of treating pain in patients receiving methadone maintenance. Similarly, their approach emphasized the need for a careful assessment with a detailed evaluation of pain and all comorbidities, appropriate analgesia with other μ-agonists added to methadone, and close monitoring by a team of professionals.

A standard approach of universal precautions incorporates ongoing evaluation of aberrant medication-taking behaviors along with monitoring the degree of analgesia, ability to perform activities of daily living, and adverse events attributable to opioid therapy [96]. The Pain Assessment and Documentation Tool operationalizes the assessment of these critical domains [26]. A recent clinical trial showed that a brief behavioral intervention utilizing urine screens, compliance checklists and motivational counseling significantly improved measures of medication misuse in patients identified as at high risk for this behavior [97]. The feeling of craving opioids is one of the most significant predictors of medication misuse and targeted by this intervention [98].

There is nothing wrong with this 'how to' algorithm, and it does imply that each step has a foundation of knowledge that must be taken into consideration. For example, a 'comprehensive evaluation' would presumably explore the patient's personal and family history of substance abuse, and an assessment of 'aberrant medication-taking behavior' would require working through a differential diagnosis as to the causes of that behavior, such as undertreatment versus addiction. The problem with these recommendations is that they are not a recipe for individual success but focus on the mechanics of prescribing opioids to the 'typical' patient.

How Do Comorbid Psychiatric Conditions Impact the Course of Chronic Pain and Opioid Dependence?

In addition to substance use disorders, other psychiatric disorders are common comorbidities of chronic pain [99–101]. The WHO reports that patients with chronic pain suffer from rates of anxiety and depressive disorders that are 4 times higher than those in patients without chronic pain [102]. These disorders are associated with an increased focus on and intensity of pain symptoms along with their associated disabilities [103]. For example, the pain arising from chronic medical disorders is rated as more severe in the presence of major depression [104]. The prevalence of psychiatric comorbidity in opioid-dependent patients receiving methadone treatment is at least 50% [105, 106]. Several pathways may result in patients with mental disorders misusing opioids, including the increased self-perception of needing more analgesics for persistent severe pain and the inappropriate self-medication for depressed and anxious emotional distress [107, 108].

In patients with chronic pain, psychiatric disorders are associated with increased rates of aberrant drug-taking behaviors and opioid use [108–110]. Psychiatric disorders are one of the most significant risk factors for being prescribed long-term opioid therapy [109, 111–113]. A prospective trial of 6,349 participants showed that common psychiatric disorders such as depression, anxiety and drug abuse disorders predict the initiation and ongoing regular use of opioids in patients with chronic pain [114].

Rates of prescription opioid use for chronic pain increase more quickly over time in patients with these disorders than in those without these disorders [115]. Similarly, a disability profile on the Minnesota Multiphasic Personality Inventory, defined as 4 or more clinical elevations or higher levels of psychopathology/emotional distress, was associated with being prescribed higher doses of opioids for the treatment of chronic pain [116].

Patients with mental disorders are also more likely to suffer from substance use disorders. The lifetime prevalence of substance use disorders in the mentally ill approaches 20% [117]. The risk of these patients using prescribed opioids is double that of those without a mental illness [114]. Similarly, the nonmedical use of opioids is associated with mood, anxiety and personality disorders [118]. The risk of developing opioid addiction is increased in patients with chronic pain who have higher levels of psychopathology [119, 120]. Conversely, over 50% of patients with substance use disorders met criteria for the diagnosis of another psychiatric disorder, with approximately one third suffering from mood disorders [121]. In studies of overdose deaths, high rates of mental illness (43%) and pain (57%) were present, and psychotropic drugs, especially benzodiazepines, contributed to half of the deaths [122].

Regardless of where this vicious cycle of comorbidity begins, the diagnosis and treatment of mental illness should be a priority in patients with chronic pain. The patient who is prescribed long-term opioid therapy is more likely to suffer from a depressive disorder, which will only compound the risk for the development of a substance use disorder. The evaluation of a patient suspected of misusing medications should be thorough and include an assessment of the pain syndrome as well as other medical disorders, patterns of medication use, social and family factors, patient and family history of substance abuse, and a comprehensive psychiatric history.

What Paradigm Exists for the Formulation and Treatment of Patients with Chronic Pain?

All mental disorders are expressions of life under altered circumstances (e.g. chronic pain) that affect characteristic mental capacities and generate particular forms of distress that will limit the effectiveness of any chronic pain treatment [123, 124]. Four perspectives (diseases, behaviors, dimensions, life stories) represent classes of disorders that each have a common essence and logical implications for causation and the treatment of emotional distress [125, 126]. In this framework of patient care, diseases are what people have, behaviors are what people do, dimensions are what people are, and life stories are what people encounter. The psychiatric formulation of any patient with chronic pain should address the contributions of each perspective to the overall presentation and inform the design of a treatment plan that can address each component of the patient's current problem list [127]. Only then will the barriers to success with interventions such as long-term opioid therapy be removed.

Diseases

Diseases of the brain manifest psychologically. The psychological faculties of the brain include, but are not limited to, consciousness, cognition, memory, language, affect and decision-making functions. Abnormalities in the structures or functions of these faculties are expressed in the criteria for mental diseases such as delirium, dementia, panic disorder and major depression. However, the patient may describe deficits in these faculties with difficulty and rely on somatic symptoms (e.g. increased or refractory pain) as incomplete proxies for these criteria. The physical symptoms occur because the brain is malfunctioning and suggesting or amplifying a pathology in the body. The unifying feature of diseases is the presence of a broken part causing a pathology [128, 129]. The pathology causes characteristic signs and symptoms typically manifested by the affliction [124]. Finding a cure may repair the broken part, prevent the initial damage from progressing, or lead to adaptation to the pathology through secondary compensatory systems. The removal of these amplifying mechanisms of chronic pain results in more effective chronic pain management that utilizes established treatment modalities.

Behaviors

The perspective of behavior encompasses a wide range of actions and activities. The complex behaviors of human beings are designed with the purpose to achieve particular goals (e.g. seeking relief from chronic pain). Internally, rhythmic alterations in attention and perception produce drives that increase a person's motivation for a particular action such as taking opioids [128, 129]. Afterwards, the drive is satisfied and a state of satiety emerges. Over time, drives reemerge with reinforcing effects on the individual's perceptual attitude towards his/her setting. In concert, personal assumptions or external opportunities increase the likelihood of certain behaviors such as repeatedly seeking consultations to determine the cause of chronic pain. Choices determine what action to take, and consequences reinforce future actions. When the choices of, and the controls over, behavior become disrupted, physicians are asked to address the distorted goals, excessive demands, damaging consequences and lack of responsiveness to negative feedback [130]. Treatment of behavioral disorders such as abnormal illness behavior begins with regaining temporary control of the situation by stopping the behavior [131, 132]. Restricting the patient's actions and preventing these problematic behaviors in a structured rehabilitative treatment program limits the chaos of destructive choices. This stable foundation is required for the patient to gain insight about, and increase his/her motivation for, appropriate choices that result in less distress and more productive behaviors [133].

Dimensions

Many mental disorders do not arise from a disease of the brain or some form of abnormal illness behavior, but from a patient's personal affective or cognitive constitution [128, 129]. Each individual possesses a set of personal dimensions such as intelligence and temperament. These traits describe who a person is and are a set of innate capabilities within his/her psychological makeup. Which traits are relied upon and how much of them a person possesses will determine his/her potential to cope with the demands of chronic pain. Some illnesses overwhelm this capacity and provoke a person's vulnerability to distress. Treatment for disorders of the dimensional type focuses on acquiring new coping skills with remediation of specific deficiencies and guidance for overcoming potential vulnerabilities, such as education about, assistance with, or modification of the particular stressors [131, 132].

Life Story
The life story perspective utilizes a narrative composed of a series of events that a person encounters and determines to be personally meaningful [128, 129]. These self-reflections are the means by which a person judges the value of his/her life as a whole. They impart a sense of self both as the agent of a life plan unfolding in a social setting, and as the reflective subject experiencing and interpreting the outcome of plans and commitments. If events unfold as planned, the person feels successful. However, if the sequence of events ends in a disappointing outcome such as suffering with chronic pain, the person feels distress over this failure. Life story disorders emerge from the negative interpretations of life encounters (grief over loss, anxiety about expected threats) [134]. Treatment forges a new understanding of settings and sequences that highlight the role of the patient in his/her life, and illuminates the troubled state of the mind as the outcome of that role and course of events [131, 132]. Effective treatment requires reframing and reinterpretation in order to remoralize the patient by transforming the story into one with the potential for future success and fulfillment. The patient with chronic pain can now envision a productive life resulting from compliance with effective treatments that limit the barriers to achieving a successful outcome.

Enhancing Treatment: New Recommendations for Integrated Approaches

Integrating specialized psychiatric treatment services (pharmacotherapies and psychotherapies) with a substance abuse treatment program is associated with significant improvement in the number of people receiving care, amount of service received, psychiatric symptoms, weekly urine test results, and self-reported ratings of response to treatment [135, 136]. This pattern of findings has also been shown in studies integrating a limited number of primary care or obstetric services into drug abuse treatment settings [137, 138]. The rationale is strong for assuming that a similar success would be achieved by the integration of on-site evaluation and treatment of chronic pain into substance abuse treatment settings managing people with opioid dependence.

A study on patients with both chronic pain and substance use disorder showed that a 10-week outpatient group therapy for pain management integrated with a multidisciplinary substance abuse treatment program was associated with a reduction in pain and emotional distress, improvement in coping skills, and a reduction in the use of pain medications including opioids [87]. The expertise of multidisciplinary pain management has largely been denied to patients with substance use disorder. Offering these patients more opioids may provide some benefits yet to be determined, but improving access to adjuvant analgesics, nonpharmacologic treatments and structured rehabilitative programs with well-documented efficacy should be a priority. At least some, and probably most, of these patients do not seek opioids merely for their intoxicating effects. An appropriate starting point assumes that patients seek relief from chronic pain and have little to no access to or knowledge of nonopioid modalities, which are clearly less controversial, potentially less destabilizing to their addiction, and likely to be more effective at decreasing pain.

Stepped-Care Treatment of Chronic Pain with Opioids in Opioid-Dependent Patients

Substance abuse treatment should utilize an adaptive yet structured treatment approach with behavioral incentives to motivate patient adherence. Many of the services constituting routine substance abuse treatment in a program with well-described outcomes, including the use of coping skills training, significant other support and incentives to increase patient adherence, are recognized as essential aspects of rehabilitative care for all people with chronic health problems including chronic pain syndromes [139–143]. Effective substance abuse therapy could indirectly benefit patients with chronic pain, attributable to the learning of new skills coupled with abstinence from drug use.

One promising approach for an integrated treatment program for chronic pain and substance use disorder involves a stepped-care strategy initially designed for routine substance abuse treatment [144–146]. The basic principle of this model of care relies on providing more services for those patients who do not meet the expectations of treatment. Patients enter treatment at a level of care that provides standard individual and group counseling, daily supervised methadone dosing, and urine screening for illicit drug use. As the patient continues treatment, additional expectations for improved function such as productive activities in the community (e.g. employment, training, volunteering), increased relationships with others who do not use drugs, and structured diversional activities are required to remain in this low intensity level of care. If the patient does well, his/her progress is reinforced by a less intensive schedule of counseling services, more flexibility in the time of methadone dosing, and increased numbers of take-home doses of methadone to reduce the number of clinic visits. Patients are motivated by the obvious positive reinforcements by methadone itself and the freedoms that result from adherence to the behavioral treatment plan. In addition, the potential for being placed in more intensive treatment with even more expectations, coupled with the loss of desired privileges, utilizes avoidance to enhance the motivation of the patients to improve their compliance with treatment.

The determination to advance a patient to more intensive treatment or a higher step of care is based on established a priori rules that utilize the results of attendance and urine testing. As a patient begins to demonstrate poor adherence to these expectations, the program adapts to that patient's individual needs. The practitioner assumes that the patient's disorder is more complex and requires more intensive treatment. Instead of being discharged from treatment because he/she is 'not ready to get well' or just trying to gain unlimited access to opioids, the patient is advanced to a higher level of care with access to more experienced senior staff, more frequent group therapy sessions, more individual counseling sessions, more closely monitored administration of methadone, and more frequent monitoring for the use of illicit drugs. If patients do not respond within a predetermined time frame, they are advanced to even higher steps of care. When patients begin responding to therapy (attend counseling sessions, decrease their use of illicit drugs), they return to less intensive treatment schedules. Increased compliance is motivated by their pursuit of desired or previously obtained positive reinforcements such as take-home doses of methadone and the opportunity to achieve or return to less restrictive schedules of care.

Patients with both chronic pain and substance dependence appear to be excellent candidates for an adaptive stepped-care treatment approach, with only minimal modifications as outlined below [147]:

1 Embrace the relationships between chronic pain and substance use disorders.
   a Inadequately treated pain causes poor adherence and response to substance abuse treatment.
   b All patients should be screened with standardized questionnaires for the presence of pain and its associated characteristics (e.g. intensity, unpleasantness, location, duration).
   c Patients should be evaluated for the impact that pain has on daily functioning and quality of life.
   d Pain-specific treatments should be initiated as soon as chronic pain disorder is discovered instead of waiting until the patient has a poor response to substance abuse treatment.
2 Expect pain to complicate substance abuse treatment.
   a Complaints of pain or signs of poor adherence should result in more aggressive diagnostic evaluation and implementation of pain management strategies (steps) that occur simultaneously with increased levels of drug abuse treatment.
   b If the pain or substance abuse problems worsen or improve independently of one another, the steps of care can be 'disconnected', with the patient, not the practitioner, determining the priority list of problems by their response to treatment.
   c The treatment should adapt to the objectively demonstrated needs of the patient and be independent from the worries or prejudices of the practitioners.

d Higher steps with more intensive treatment must still offer to the patient a doable set of changes to the treatment plan.

e The efficacy of the step must be assessed for all patients in order to determine whether the content of that treatment step is adequate or whether additional steps of even more intensive treatment are required for the most complex patients.

3 Maximize the benefits of methadone, the analgesic properties of which have limited duration.

a Consider increasing the total daily dose to enhance analgesia.

b Consider utilizing a split-dose or b.i.d. dosing schedule to increase the duration of analgesia.

c Earning take-home doses can facilitate implementing an every-6-hour dosing schedule for incremental improvement in the duration of analgesia.

4 Introduce nonopioid therapies early.

a The use of nonopioid therapies for chronic pain is inexcusably rare.

b Education about and group therapy concerning the efficacy of nonopioid medications and nonpharmacological modalities of managing chronic pain should be provided.

c Stress management, coping skills training, relaxation/biofeedback techniques and physical therapies directed at reducing chronic pain and improving function should be utilized.

d Higher steps of pain management should offer more individual sessions to understand and address the problems likely to be more specific to the refractory patient.

e Medications such as antidepressants and anticonvulsants used to treat neuropathic pain should be prescribed.

f If necessary, the dosing of these medications may be monitored in conjunction with their methadone and administered under observation by program staff to insure the medication is taken as prescribed.

g Serum levels may be obtained to monitor compliance as well as adjust dosing schedules.

Conclusions and Future Research

As noted at the outset of this review, one of the more important aspects of successful management of patients with both chronic pain and substance use disorder is avoiding the trap of deciding whether complaints of pain are 'real' or a manifestation of 'drug seeking'. This trap leads to a premature and informed guess about the need to focus treatment on either pain or substance abuse. The initial assumption is simple. Their complaints of pain are real, and not a manifestation of substance abuse but a request for treatment. Until is it clear just what forms of treatment should be utilized, treatment should address both problems simultaneously. Patients should be initiated into therapy with a comprehensive evaluation of the characteristics and severity of their specific problems. If more than one problem exists, a multidisciplinary treatment plan should be formulated.

The patient's ongoing response to treatment for each problem should be frequently assessed. The problem-specific outcome measures should then guide the degree to which each problem receives more intensive therapy. Despite best intentions, this approach usually devolves to an excessive focus on one problem coupled with an inadequate focus on the other problem. First, it is crucial to remember patients have both problems, and both disorders require ongoing careful evaluation. Second, an ongoing discussion with patients and family about their response to treatment should occur regularly. Finally, how the continuing plan of care will be modified should be clear to all parties. These basic principles of treatment form the foundation for a program designed to motivate patients in treatment and adapt to individual needs to insure successful outcomes.

References

1 Fleming M, Balousek S, Klessig C, Mundt M, Brown D: Substance use disorders in a primary care sample receiving daily opioid therapy. J Pain 2007;8:573–582.
2 Rosenblum A, Joseph H, Fong C, Kipnis S, Cleland C, Portenoy RK: Prevalence and characteristics of chronic pain among chemically dependent patients in methadone maintenance and residential treatment facilities. JAMA 2003;289:2370–2378.
3 Peles E, Schreiber S, Gordon J, Adelson M: Significantly higher methadone dose for methadone maintenance treatment (MMT) patients with chronic pain. Pain 2005;113:340–346.
4 Nickel R, Raspe HH: Chronic pain: epidemiology and health care utilization (in German). Nervenarzt 2001;72:897–906.
5 Ospina M, Harstall C: Prevalence of chronic pain: an overview. Health Technology Assessment Report No 29. 2002. http://www.ihe.ca/hta/publications.html.
6 Verhaak PF, Kerssens JJ, Dekker J, Sorbi MJ, Bensing JM: Prevalence of chronic benign pain disorder among adults: a review of the literature. Pain 1998;77:231–239.
7 Elliott AM, Smith BH, Hannaford PC, Smith WC, Chambers WA: The course of chronic pain in the community: results of a 4-year follow-up study. Pain 2002;99:299–307.
8 Mäntyselkä PT, Turunen JH, Ahonen RS, Kumpusalo EA: Chronic pain and poor self-rated health. JAMA 2003;290:2435–2442.
9 Stewart WF, Ricci JA, Chee E, Morganstein D, Lipton R: Lost productive time and cost due to common pain conditions in the US workforce. JAMA 2003;290:2443–2454.
10 Brands B, Blake J, Sproule B, Gourlay D, Busto U: Prescription opioid abuse in patients presenting for methadone maintenance treatment. Drug Alcohol Depend 2004;73:199–207.
11 Dowling LS, Gatchel RJ, Adams LL, Stowell AW, Bernstein D: An evaluation of the predictive validity of the Pain Medication Questionnaire with a heterogeneous group of patients with chronic pain. J Opioid Manag 2007;3:257–266.
12 Mertens JR, Lu YW, Parthasarathy S, Moore C, Weisner CM: Medical and psychiatric conditions of alcohol and drug treatment patients in an HMO: comparison with matched controls. Arch Intern Med 2003;163:2511–2517.
13 Portenoy RK, Dole V, Joseph H, Lowinson J, Rice C, Segal S, Richman BL: Pain management and chemical dependency: evolving perspectives. JAMA 1997;278:592–593.
14 Scimeca MM, Savage SR, Portenoy R, Lowinson J: Treatment of pain in methadone-maintained patients. Mt Sinai J Med 2000;67:412–422.
15 Cohen MJ, Jasser S, Herron PD, Margolis CG: Ethical perspectives: opioid treatment of chronic pain in the context of addiction. Clin J Pain 2002;18(suppl 4):S99–S107.

16 Drug Enforcement Administration: A joint statement from 21 health organizations and the Drug Enforcement Administration. Promoting pain relief and preventing abuse of pain medications: a critical balancing act. J Pain Symptom Manage 2002;24:147.

17 Nicholson B: Responsible prescribing of opioids for the management of chronic pain. Drugs 2003;63: 17–32.

18 Trafton JA, Oliva EM, Horst DA, Minkel JD, Humphreys K: Treatment needs associated with pain in substance use disorder patients: implications for concurrent treatment. Drug Alcohol Depend 2004;73:23–31.

19 Compton P, Darakjian J, Miotto K: Screening for addiction in patients with chronic pain and 'problematic' substance use: evaluation of a pilot assessment tool. J Pain Symptom Manage 1998;16:355–363.

20 Miotto K, Compton P, Ling W, Conolly M: Diagnosing addictive disease in chronic pain patients. Psychosomatics 1996;37:223–235.

21 Robinson RC, Gatchel RJ, Polatin P, Deschner M, Noe C, Gajraj N: Screening for problematic prescription opioid use. Clin J Pain 2001;17:220–228.

22 Savage SR: Assessment for addiction in pain-treatment settings. Clin J Pain 2002;18:S28–S38.

23 Højsted J, Sjøgren P: Addiction to opioids in chronic pain patients: a literature review. Eur J Pain 2007;11: 490–518.

24 Portenoy RK: Opioid therapy for chronic nonmalignant pain: a review of the critical issues. J Pain Symptom Manage 1996;11:203–217.

25 Passik SD, Kirsh KL: Managing pain in patients with aberrant drug-taking behaviors. J Support Oncol 2005;3:83–86.

26 Passik SD, Kirsh KL, Whitcomb L, Schein JR, Kaplan MA, Dodd SL, Kleinman L, Katz NP, Portenoy RK: Monitoring outcomes during long-term opioid therapy for noncancer pain: results with the Pain Assessment and Documentation Tool. J Opioid Manag 2005;1:257–266.

27 Portenoy RK: Appropriate use of opioids for persistent non-cancer pain. Lancet 2004;364:739–740.

28 Savage SR: Addiction in the treatment of pain: significance, recognition and management. J Pain Symptom Manage 1993;8:265–278.

29 Sees KL, Clark HW: Opioid use in the treatment of chronic pain: assessment of addiction. J Pain Symptom Manage 1993;8:257–264.

30 Cicero TJ, Dart RC, Inciardi JA, Woody GE, Schnoll S, Muñoz A: The development of a comprehensive risk-management program for prescription opioid analgesics: Researched Abuse, Diversion and Addiction-Related Surveillance (RADARS). Pain Med 2007;8:157–170.

31 Olsen Y, Daumit GL, Ford DE: Opioid prescriptions by US primary care physicians from 1992 to 2001. J Pain 2006;7:223–235.

32 Gilson AM, Ryan KM, Joranson DE, Dahl JL: A reassessment of trends in the medical use and abuse of opioid analgesics and implications for diversion control: 1997–2002. J Pain Symptom Manage 2004; 28:176–188.

33 Cicero TJ, Inciardi JA, Muñoz A: Trends in abuse of OxyContin and other opioid analgesics in the United States: 2002–2004. J Pain 2005;6:662–672.

34 Cicero TJ, Inciardi JA, Surratt H: Trends in the use and abuse of branded and generic extended release oxycodone and fentanyl products in the United States. Drug Alcohol Depend 2007;91:115–120.

35 Lamb E: Top 200 prescription drugs of 2007. Pharm Times 2008;74:20–23.

36 Smith MY, Schneider MF, Wentz A, Hughes A, Haddox JD, Dart R: Quantifying morbidity associated with the abuse and misuse of opioid analgesics: a comparison of two approaches. Clin Toxicol 2007; 45:23–30.

37 Cicero TJ, Inciardi JA: Diversion and abuse of methadone prescribed for pain management. JAMA 2005;293:297–298.

38 Brown RL, Patterson JJ, Rounds LA, Papasouliotis O: Substance abuse among patients with chronic back pain. J Fam Pract 1996;43:152–160.

39 Aronoff GM: Opioids in chronic pain management: is there a significant risk of addiction? Curr Rev Pain 2000;4:112–121.

40 Fishbain D, Cutler R, Rosomoff H: Comorbid psychiatric disorders in chronic pain patients. Pain Clin 1998;11:79–87.

41 Portenoy RK, Foley KM: Chronic use of opioid analgesics in non-malignant pain: report of 38 cases. Pain 1986;25:171–186.

42 Taub A: Opioid analgesics in the treatment of chronic intractable pain on non-neoplastic origin; in Kitahata LM, Collins D (eds): Narcotic Analgesics in Anesthesiology. Baltimore, Williams and Wilkins, 1982, pp 199–208.

43 Jamison RN, Kauffman J, Katz NP: Characteristics of methadone maintenance patients with chronic pain. J Pain Symptom Manage 2000;19:53–62.

44 Larson MJ, Paasche-Orlow M, Cheng DM, Lloyd-Travaglini C, Saitz R, Samet JH: Persistent pain is associated with substance use after detoxification: a prospective cohort analysis. Addiction 2007;102: 752–760.

45 Fishbain DA, Cole B, Lewis J, Rosomoff HL, Rosomoff RS: What percentage of chronic nonmalignant pain patients exposed to chronic opioid analgesic therapy develop abuse/addiction and/or aberrant drug-related behaviors? A structured evidence-based review. Pain Med 2008;9:444–459.

46 Moore TM, Jones T, Browder JH, Daffron S, Passik SD: A comparison of common screening methods for predicting aberrant drug-related behavior among patients receiving opioids for chronic pain management. Pain Med 2009;10:1426–1433.

47 Michna E, Ross EL, Hynes WL, Nedeljkovic SS, Soumekh S, Janfaza D, Palombi D, Jamison RN: Predicting aberrant drug behavior in patients treated for chronic pain: importance of abuse history. J Pain Symptom Manage 2004;28:250–258.

48 Højsted J, Nielsen PR, Guldstrand SK, Frich L, Sjøgren P: Classification and identification of opioid addiction in chronic pain patients. Eur J Pain 2010;14:1014–1020.

49 Kirsh KL, Whitcomb LA, Donaghy K, Passik SD: Abuse and addiction issues in medically ill patients with pain: attempts at clarification of terms and empirical study. Clin J Pain 2002;18:S52–S60.

50 Weaver M, Schnoll S: Abuse liability in opioid therapy for pain treatment in patients with an addiction history. Clin J Pain 2002;18:S61–S69.

51 Potter JS, Hennessy G, Borrow JA, Greenfield SF, Weiss RD: Substance use histories in patients seeking treatment for controlled-release oxycodone dependence. Drug Alcohol Depend 2004;76:213–215.

52 Eisenberg E, McNicol ED, Carr DB: Efficacy and safety of opioid agonists in the treatment of neuropathic pain of nonmalignant origin: systematic review and meta-analysis of randomized controlled trials. JAMA 2005;293:3043–3052.

53 Furlan AD, Sandoval JA, Mallis-Gagnon A, Tunks E: Opioids for chronic noncancer pain: a meta-analysis of effectiveness and side effects. Can Med Assoc J 2006;174:1589–1594.

54 Noble M, Tregear SJ, Treadwell JR, Schoelles K: Long-term opioid therapy for chronic noncancer pain: a systematic review and meta-analysis of efficacy and safety. J Pain Symptom Manage 2008;35:214–228.

55 Devulder J, Richarz U, Nataraja SH: Impact of long-term use of opioids on quality of life in patients with chronic nonmalignant pain. Curr Med Res Opin 2005;84:S42–S55.

56 Ballantyne JC, Mao J: Opioid therapy for chronic pain. N Engl J Med 2003;349:1943–1953.

57 Eriksen J, Sjøgren P, Bruera E, Ekholm O, Rasmussen NK: Critical issues on opioids in chronic non-cancer pain: an epidemiological study. Pain 2006;125:172–179.

58 Fields HL: Should we be reluctant to prescribe opioids for chronic non-malignant pain? Pain 2007;129:233–234.

59 Kalso E, Edwards JE, Moore RA, McQuay HJ: Opioids in chronic non-cancer pain: systematic review of efficacy and safety. Pain 2004;112:372–380.

60 Franklin GM, Mai J, Wickizer T, Turner JA, Fulton-Kehoe D, Grant L: Opioid dosing trends and mortality in Washington State workers' compensation, 1996–2002. Am J Ind Med 2005;48:91–99.

61 Chou R, Fanciullo GJ, Fine PG, Miaskowski C, Passik SD, Portenoy RK: Opioids for chronic noncancer pain: prediction and identification of aberrant drug-related behaviors – a review of the evidence for an American Pain Society and American Academy of Pain Medicine clinical practice guideline. J Pain 2009;10:131–146.

62 Passik SD, Kirsh KL, Donaghy KB, Portenoy RK: Pain and aberrant drug-related behaviors in medically ill patients with and without histories of substance abuse. Clin J Pain 2006;22:173–181.

63 von Korff M, Saunders K, Thomas Ray G, Boudreau D, Campbell C, Merrill J, Sullivan MD, Rutter CM, Silverberg MJ, Banta-Green C, Weisner C: De facto long-term opioid therapy for noncancer pain. Clin J Pain 2008;24:521–527.

64 McCracken LM, Hoskins J, Eccleston C: Concerns about medication and medication use in chronic pain. J Pain 2006;7:726–734.

65 Schieffer BM, Pham Q, Labus J, Baria A, van Vort W, Davis P, Davis F, Naliboff BD: Pain medication beliefs and medication misuse in chronic pain. J Pain 2005;6:620–629.

66 Karasz A, Zallman L, Berg K, Gourevitch M, Selwyn P, Amsten JH: The experience of chronic severe pain in patients undergoing methadone maintenance treatment. J Pain Symptom Manage 2004;28:517–525.

67 Sullivan MD, von Korff M, Banta-Green C, Merrill JO, Saunders K: Problems and concerns of patients receiving chronic opioid therapy for chronic noncancer pain. Pain 2010;149:345–353.

68 Noble M, Treadwell JR, Tregear SJ, Coates VH, Wiffen PJ, Akafomo C, Schoelles KM: Long-term opioid management for chronic noncancer pain. Cochrane Database Syst Rev 2010;20:CD006605.

69 Dworkin RH, Turk DC, Wyrwich KW, Beaton D, Cleeland CS, Farrar JT, Haythornthwaite JA, Jensen MP, Kerns RD, Ader DN, Brandenburg N, Burke LB, Cella D, Chandler J, Cowan P, Dimitrova R, Dionne R, Hertz S, Jadad AR, Katz NP, Kehlet H, Kramer LD, Manning DC, McCormick C, McDermott MP, McQuay HJ, Patel S, Porter L, Quessy S, Rappaport BA, Rauschkolb C, Revicki DA, Rothman M, Schmader KE, Stacey BR, Stauffer JW, von Stein T, White RE, Witter J, Zavisic S: Interpreting the clinical importance of treatment outcomes in chronic pain clinical trials: impact recommendations. J Pain 2008;9:105–121.

70 Pflughaupt M, Scharnagel R, Gossrau G, Kaiser U, Koch T, Sabatowski R: Physicians' knowledge and attitudes concerning the use of opioids in the treatment of chronic cancer and non-cancer pain (in German). Schmerz 2010;24:267–275.

71 Wolfert MZ, Gilson AM, Dahl JL, Cleary JF: Opioid analgesics for pain control: Wisconsin physicians' knowledge, beliefs, attitudes, and prescribing practices. Pain Med 2010;11:425–434.

72 Upshur CC, Luckmann RS, Savageau JA: Primary care provider concerns about management of chronic pain in community clinic populations. J Gen Intern Med 2006;21:652–655.

73 Wasan AD, Correll DJ, Kissin I, O'Shea S, Jamison RN: Iatrogenic addiction in patients treated for acute or subacute pain: a systematic review. J Opioid Manag 2006;2:16–22.

74 Gilson AM, Maurer MA, Joranson DE: State medical board members' beliefs about pain, addiction, and diversion and abuse: a changing regulatory environment. J Pain 2007;8:682–691.

75 Breivik H, Collett B, Ventafridda V, Cohen R, Gallacher D: Survey of chronic pain in Europe: prevalence, impact on daily life, and treatment. Eur J Pain 2006;10:287–333.

76 Galvez R: Variable use of opioid pharmacotherapy for chronic noncancer pain in Europe: causes and consequences. J Pain Palliat Care Pharmacother 2009;23:346–356.

77 Ziegler SJ, Lovrich NP: Pain relief, prescription drugs, and prosecution: a four-state survey of chief prosecutors. J Law Med Ethics 2003;31:75–100.

78 Haller DL, Acosta MC: Characteristics of pain patients with opioid-use disorder. Psychosomatics 2010;51:257–266.

79 Baldacchino A, Gilchrist G, Fleming R, Bannister J: Guilty until proven innocent: a qualitative study of the management of chronic non-cancer pain among patients with a history of substance abuse. Addict Behav 2010;35:270–272.

80 Chapman CR, Lipschitz DL, Angst MS, Chou R, Denisco RC, Donaldson GW, Fine PG, Foley KM, Gallagher RM, Gilson AM, Haddox JD, Horn SD, Inturrisi CE, Jick SS, Lipman AG, Loeser JD, Noble M, Porter L, Rowbotham MC, Schoelles KM, Turk DC, Volinn E, von Korff MR, Webster LF, Weisner CM: Opioid pharmacotherapy for chronic noncancer pain in the United States: a research guideline for developing an evidence-base. J Pain 2010;11: 807–829.

81 Harris JM Jr, Elliott TE, Davis BE, Chabal C, Fulginiti JV, Pine PG: Educating generalist physicians about chronic pain: live experts and online education can provide durable benefits. Pain Med 2008;9:555–563.

82 Harris JM Jr, Fulginiti JV, Gordon PR, Elliott TE, Davis BE, Chabal C, Kutob RM: KnowPain-50: a tool for assessing physician pain management education. Pain Med 2008;9:542–554.

83 Passik SD: Issues in long-term opioid therapy: unmet needs, risks, and solutions. Mayo Clin Proc 2009;84:593–601.

84 Ehde DM, Jensen MP, Engel JM, Turner JA, Hoffman AJ, Cardenas DD: Chronic pain secondary to disability: a review. Clin J Pain 2003;19: 3–17.

85 Foley K: Pain in the elderly; in Hazzard WR, Bierman EL, Blass JP, Ettinger W, Halter J (eds): Principles of Geriatric Medicine and Gerontology, ed 3. New York, McGraw-Hill, 1994, pp 126–149.

86 Gordon RS: Pain in the elderly. JAMA 1979;241: 2191–2192.

87 Currie SR, Hodgins DC, Crabtree A, Jacobi J, Armstrong SJ: Outcome from integrated pain management treatment for recovering substance abusers. Pain 2003;4:91–100.

88 Fuller CM, Borrell LN, Latkin CA, Galea S, Ompad DC, Strathdee SA, Vlohov D: Effects of race, neighborhood, and social network on age at initiation of injection drug use. Am J Public Health 2005;95: 689–695.

89 Kidorf M, Brooner RK: Special section – the most critical unresolved issues associated with contemporary vocational rehabilitation for substance users: the critical relationship between employment services and patient motivation. Subst Use Misuse 2004;39:2611–2614.

90 Kidorf M, Brooner RK, King VL, Stoller KB, Wertz J: Predictive validity of cocaine, benzodiazepine, and alcohol dependence diagnoses. J Consult Clin Psychol 1998;66:168–173.

91 Kidorf M, Disney ER, King VL, Neufeld K, Beilenson PL, Brooner RK: Prevalence of psychiatric and substance use disorders in opioid abusers in a community syringe exchange program. Drug Alcohol Depend 2004;74:115–122.

92 Kidorf M, Neufeld K, Brooner RK: Combining stepped-care approaches with behavioral reinforcement to motivate employment in opioid-dependent outpatients. Subst Use Misuse 2004;39: 2215–2238.

93 Kidorf M, King VL, Neufeld K, Stoller KB, Peirce J, Brooner RK: Involving significant others in the care of opioid-dependent patients receiving methadone. J Subst Abuse Treat 2005;29:19–27.

94 Chou R, Fanciullo GJ, Fine PG, Adler JA, Ballantyne JC, Davies P, Donovan MI, Fishbain DA, Foley KM, Fudin J, Gilson AM, Kelter A, Mauskop A, O'Connor PG, Passik SD, Pasternak GW, Portenoy RK, Rich BA, Roberts RG, Todd KH, Miaskowski C, American Pain Society-American Academy of Pain Medicine Opioids Guidelines Panel: Clinical guidelines for the use of chronic opioid therapy in chronic noncancer pain. J Pain 2009;10:113–130.

95 Manchikanti L, Benyamin R, Datta S, Vallejo R, Smith H: Opioids in chronic noncancer pain. Expert Rev Neurother 2010;10:775–789.

96 Smith HS, Kirsh KL, Passik SD: Chronic opioid therapy issues associated with opioid abuse potential. J Opioid Manag 2009;5:287–300.

97 Jamison RN, Butler SF, Budman SH, Edwards RR, Wasan AD: Gender differences in risk factors for aberrant prescription opioid use. J Pain 2010;11: 312–320.

98 Wasan AD, Butler SF, Budman SH, Fernandez K, Weiss RD, Greenfield S, Jamison RN: Does report of craving opioid medication predict aberrant drug behavior among chronic pain patients? Clin J Pain 2009;25:193–198.

99 Dersh J, Polatin PB, Gatchel RJ: Chronic pain and psychopathology: research findings and theoretical considerations. Psychosom Med 2002;64:773–786.

100 Fishbain DA, Goldberg M, Meagher BR, Steele R, Rosomoff H: Male and female chronic pain patients categorized by DSM-III psychiatric diagnostic criteria. Pain 1986;26:181–197.

101 Harter M, Reuter K, Weisser B, Schretzmann B, Aschenbrenner A, Bengel J: A descriptive study of psychiatric disorders and psychosocial burden in rehabilitation patients with musculoskeletal diseases. Arch Phys Med Rehabil 2002;83:461–468.

102 Gureje O, Simon GE, von Korff M: A cross-national study of the course of persistent pain in primary care. Pain 2001;92:195–200.

103 Bair MJ, Wu J, Damush TM, Sutherland JM, Kroenke K: Association of depression and anxiety alone and in combination with chronic musculoskeletal pain in primary care patients. Psychosom Med 2008;70:890–897.

104 Katon W, Sullivan M, Walker E: Medical symptoms without identified pathology: relationship to psychiatric disorders, childhood and adult trauma and personality traits. Ann Intern Med 2001;134: 917–925.

105 Brooner RK, King VL, Kidorf M, Schmidt CW, Bigelow GE: Psychiatric and substance use comorbidity among treatment-seeking opioid abusers. Arch Gen Psychiatry 1997;54:71–80.

106 Khantzian EJ, Treece C: DSM-III psychiatric diagnosis of narcotic addicts. Arch Gen Psychiatry 1985; 42:1067–1071.

107 Geisser ME, Cano A, Foran H: Psychometric properties of the mood and anxiety symptom questionnaire in patients with chronic pain. Clin J Pain 2006; 22:1–9.

108 Wasan AD, Butler SF, Budman SH, Benoit C, Fernandez K, Jamison RN: Psychiatric history and psychological adjustment as risk factors for aberrant drug-related behavior among patients with chronic pain. Clin J Pain 2007;23:307–315.

109 Sullivan MD, Edlund MJ, Steffick D, Unützer J: Regular use of prescribed opioids: association with common psychiatric disorders. Pain 2005;119: 95–103.

110 Manchikanti L, Giordano J, Boswell M, Fellows B, Manchukonda R, Pampati V: Psychological factors as predictors of opioid abuse and illicit drug use in chronic pain patients. J Opioid Manag 2007;3: 89–100.

111 Reid MC, Engles-Horton LL, Weber MB, Kerns RD, Rogers EL, O'Connor PG: Use of opioid medications for chronic noncancer pain syndromes in primary care. J Gen Intern Med 2002;17:173–179.

112 Breckenridge J, Clark JD: Patient characteristics associated with opioid versus nonsteroidal anti-inflammatory drug management of chronic low back pain. J Pain 2003;4:344–350.

113 Braden JB, Sullivan MD, Ray GT, Saunders K, Merrill J, Silverberg MJ, Rutter CM, Weisner C, Banta-Green C, Campbell C, von Korff M: Trends in long-term opioid therapy for noncancer pain among persons with a history of depression. Gen Hosp Psychiatry 2009;31:564–570.

114 Sullivan MD, Edlund MJ, Zhang L, Unützer J, Wells KB: Association between mental health disorders, problem drug use, and regular prescription opioid use. Arch Intern Med 2006;166: 2087–2093.

115 Edlund MJ, Martin BC, Devries A, Fan MY, Braden JB, Sullivan MD: Trends in use of opioids for chronic noncancer pain among individuals with mental health and substance use disorders: the TROUP study. Clin J Pain 2010;26:1–8.

116 Kidner CL, Gatchel RJ, Mayer TG: MMPI disability profile is associated with degree of opioid use in chronic work-related musculoskeletal disorders. Clin J Pain 2010;26:9–15.

117 Hasin DS, Goodwin RD, Stinson FS, Grant BF: Epidemiology of major depressive disorder: results from the National Epidemiologic Survey on Alcoholism and Related Conditions. Arch Gen Psychiatry 2005;62:1097–1106.

118 Huang B, Dawson DA, Stinson FS, Hasin DS, Ruan WJ, Saha TD, Smith SM, Goldstein RB, Grant BF: Prevalence, correlates, and comorbidity of nonmedical prescription drug use and drug use disorders in the United States: results of the National Epidemiologic Survey on Alcohol and Related Conditions. J Clin Psychiatry 2006;67: 1062–1073.

119 Nedeljkovic SS, Wasan A, Jamison RN: Assessment of efficacy of long-term opioid therapy in pain patients with substance abuse potential. Clin J Pain 2002;18:S39–S51.

120 Strain EC: Assessment and treatment of comorbid psychiatric disorders in opioid-dependent patients. Clin J Pain 2002;18:S14–S27.

121 Grant BF, Stinson FS, Dawson DA, Chou SP, Dufour MC, Compton W, Pickering RP, Kaplan K: Prevalence and co-occurrence of substance use disorders and independent mood and anxiety disorders: results from the National Epidemiologic Survey on Alcohol and Related Conditions. Arch Gen Psychiatry 2004;61:807–816.

122 Toblin RL, Paulozzi LJ, Logan JE, Hall AJ, Kaplan JA: Mental illness and psychotropic drug use among prescription drug overdose deaths: a medical examiner chart review. J Clin Psychiatry 2010;71: 491–496.

123 Brown RJ: Psychological mechanisms of medically unexplained symptoms: an integrative conceptual model. Psychol Bull 2004;130:793–812.

124 Rief W, Barsky AJ: Psychobiological perspectives on somatoform disorders. Psychoneuroendocrinology 2005;30:996–1002.

125 McHugh PR, Slavney PR: Methods of reasoning in psychopathology: conflict and resolution. Compr Psychiatry 1982;23:197–215.

126 McHugh PR: A structure for psychiatry at the century's turn: the view from Johns Hopkins. J R Soc Med 1992;85:483–487.

127 Clark MR: Psychiatry and chronic pain: examining the interface and designing a structure for a patient-centered approach to treatment. Eur J Pain 2009; 13(suppl):95–100.

128 McHugh PR, Slavney PR: Perspectives of Psychiatry, ed 2. Baltimore, Johns Hopkins University Press, 1998.

129 Slavney PR: Perspectives on 'Hysteria'. Baltimore, Johns Hopkins University Press, 1990.

130 Reuber M, Mitchell AJ, Howlett SJ, Crimlisk HL, Grunewald RA: Functional symptoms in neurology: questions and answers. J Neurol Neurosurg Psychiatry 2005;76:307–314.

131 Clark MR: Psychogenic disorders: a pragmatic approach for formulation and treatment. Sem Neurol 2006;26:357–365.

132 Clark MR, Treisman GJ: Perspectives on pain and depression. Adv Psychosom Med 2004;25:1–27.

133 Stone J, Carson A, Sharpe M: Functional symptoms and signs in neurology: management. J Neurol Neurosurg Psychiatry 2005;76(suppl 1): i13–i21.

134 Rief W, Nanke A: Somatoform disorders in primary care and inpatient settings. Adv Psychosom Med 2004;26:144–158.

135 King VL, Peirce J, Brooner RK, Kidorf M: Predictors of treatment enrollment in syringe exchange participants. Presented at College on Problems of Drug Dependence Scientific Meeting, Quebec City, 2007.

136 Brooner RK, King V, Neufeld K, Stoller K, Peirce J, Kidorf M, Clark M, Aklin W: Integrated psychiatric services are associated with improved service delivery and better treatment response. Presented at College on Problems of Drug Dependence 70th Annual Scientific Meeting, San Juan, 2008.

137 Umbricht-Schneiter A, Ginn DH, Pabst KM, Bigelow GE: Providing medical care to methadone clinic patients: referral vs on-site care. Am J Public Health 1994;84:207–210.

138 Svikis DS, Silverman K, Hauq NA, Stitzer M, Keyser-Marcus L: Behavioral strategies to improve treatment participation and retention by pregnant drug-dependent women. Subst Use Misuse 2007;42: 1527–1535.

139 Flor H, Fydrich T, Turk DC: Efficacy of multidisciplinary pain treatment centers: a meta-analytic review. Pain 1992;49:221–230.

140 Haythornthwaite JA: Clinical trials studying pharmacotherapy and psychological treatments alone and together. Neurology 2005;65:20–31.

141 Maruta T, Malinchoc M, Offord KP, Colligan RC: Status of patients with chronic pain 13 years after treatment in a pain management center. Pain 1998; 74:199–204.

142 Morley S, Eccleston C, Williams A: Systematic review and meta-analysis of randomized controlled trials of cognitive behaviour therapy and behaviour therapy for chronic pain in adults, excluding headache. Pain 1999;80:1–13.

143 Turk DC, Okifuji A: Psychological factors in chronic pain: evolution and revolution. J Consult Clin Psychol 2002;70:678–690.

144 Brooner RK, Kidorf M: Using behavioral reinforcement to improve methadone treatment participation. Sci Pract Perspect 2002;1:38–46.

145 Brooner RK, Kidorf MS, King VL, Stoller KB, Peirce JM, Bigelow GE, Kolodner K: Behavioral contingencies improve counseling attendance in an adaptive treatment model. J Subst Abuse Treat 2004; 27:223–232.

146 Brooner RK, Kidorf MS, King VL, Stoller KB, Neufeld KJ, Kolodner K: Comparing adaptive stepped care and monetary-based voucher incentives for opioid dependence. Drug Alcohol Depend 2007;88(suppl 2):S14–S23.

147 Clark MR, Stoller KB, Brooner RK: Assessment and management of chronic pain in individuals seeking treatment for opioid dependence disorder. Can J Psychiatry 2008;53:496–508.

Michael R. Clark, MD, MPH
Department of Psychiatry and Behavioral Sciences
Osler 320, The Johns Hopkins Hospital, 600 North Wolfe Street
Baltimore, MD 21287-5371 (USA)
Tel. +1 410 955 2126, E-Mail mclark9@jhmi.edu

Clark MR, Treisman GJ (eds): Chronic Pain and Addiction.
Adv Psychosom Med. Basel, Karger, 2011, vol 30, pp 113–124

Screening for Abuse Risk in Pain Patients

Tara M. Bohn · Lauren B. Levy · Sheyla Celin · Tatiana D. Starr ·
Steven D. Passik

Department of Psychiatry and Behavioral Sciences, Memorial Sloan-Kettering Cancer Center,
New York, N.Y., USA

Abstract

As opioid prescribing has dramatically expanded over the past decade, so too has the problem of prescription drug abuse. In response to these now two major public health problems – the problem of poorly treated chronic pain and the problem of opioid abuse – a new paradigm has arisen in pain management, namely risk stratification. Once a prescriber has determined that opioids will be used (a medical decision based on how intense the pain is, what has been tried and failed and, to some extent, what type of pain the patient has), he/she must then decide how opioid therapy is to be delivered. Different models of delivery of opioid therapy can be utilized, beginning the process with a risk assessment that is highly individualized to each patient. Recently, researchers have produced a wide variety of literature regarding assessment tools to be used for this purpose. And while there remains a need for larger prospective studies to examine the ability of each tool to predict aberrant drug-taking behaviors, clinicians can and should utilize one or more of these screening tools and understand their benefits and limitations. This chapter will describe the nature of current screening assessments, their potential for use in the pain population in various settings, past clinical observations and suggestions for moving forward.

Millions of Americans are impacted by chronic pain, a major health concern in the USA that not only reduces productivity among the population, but also undermines their quality of life. Depression, anxiety and sleep disturbance are among the many physical and psychological comorbidities which patients experience [1]. Despite advancement in pain treatment and management, chronic pain continues to be problematic due to a variety of complicating factors.

Healthcare providers are often reluctant to address the concerns of pain patients for a number of reasons. Treatment of chronic pain can be complex and requires a multidisciplinary approach, which is becoming increasingly difficult to provide due to poor reimbursement from managed care organizations. Practitioners may be skeptical of a patient that lacks the objective signs of physiological stress. Prescription drug abuse and a hostile regulatory climate have caused clinicians to shy away from prescribing opioids, especially to patients who have a history of abuse, suggesting a greater risk for repeat abuse [2, 3].

However, the paradigm of long-term opioid therapy has shifted from past stigmas and fear of opioid use to an emphasis on the importance of finding a balance between safety and effectiveness in treatment. Both undertreated pain and aberrant drug-related behavior have become significant public health problems. The clinical community must adopt risk assessment and monitoring practices in order to enforce a universal standard of optimal treatment. It is crucial that prescribers utilize risk assessment tools in addition to their clinical judgment to guide them toward the most appropriate treatment regimen for a particular patient. As such, many instruments have been designed to help screen for abuse risk in pain patients being considered for opioid therapy. The use of assessment tools fulfills the requirement for due diligence in the areas of screening for the patient's vulnerabilities and incorporating the results of these assessments into treatment planning. Additionally, the use of validated tools not only helps guide the assessment, but when incorporated into the medical record, also upgrades the clinician's documentation of this assessment.

Pain and Substance Abuse

The USA has seen a substantial increase in prescriptions of pain medicines, although chronic pain remains poorly treated [4]. There has been a wider availability of opioids, which has created larger concern about abuse. To illustrate, 9.4 billion doses of opioids were consumed from 2002 to 2005, and 190 million opioid prescriptions were written during this time [5]. According to the SAMHSA (Substance Abuse and Mental Health Services Administration), opioids became the new drug of choice, displacing marijuana for the very first time. In addition, the National Survey on Drug Use and Health data reported at least 430 million doses abused in 2006 [6]. Clinicians rationalize that although opioids are effective, there is potential for drug abuse and diversion. Unlike prescription of any other medication class, prescription of opioids requires a treatment agreement or documentation of informed consent.

Proper assessments should be performed to identify patients with genuine pain, those who may or may not be using their medications properly, as well as those who exaggerate their pain to gain access to opioids. Chronic pain assessment should detail the intensity, quality, location and radiation of pain. Additionally, the evaluation should identify the factors that increase and decrease the pain, as well as review the effectiveness of all interventions that have been tried to relieve pain.

Pain Assessment

The influence of pain on sleep, temperament, stress levels, function at work, relationships and recreation should be assessed as these areas may be influenced by pain treatment. In addition, the presence of baseline scores prior to administering an intervention can help clinicians measure the effectiveness of treatments. There are already a number of general pain screening instruments, such as the Brief Pain Inventory, that were developed to help assess these areas [7–9]. While these tools have proven useful for a generalized assessment of pain, additional measures must be employed to examine the potential risk of aberrant behavior.

The following is a compilation of many of the available risk assessment instruments for opioid abuse. Although not a complete answer, this list can help physicians determine if they are within or outside the guidelines of peer-approved prescribing methods. The descriptions of each measure include details regarding their mode, ease of administration, psychometric properties and target population, as well as the aspects of addiction that each tool is designed to monitor or predict.

Screening Tools for Pain Populations

Atluri Screening Tool

Atluri and Sudarshan [10] developed a clinician-rated screening tool to detect the risk of questionable opioid use in patients with chronic pain. The authors identified 6 clinical criteria considered demonstrative of opioid abuse. Evaluation of the 6 criteria is reviewed by the screening tool through a checklist of questions. Patients respond 'yes' or 'no' to items related to opioids, opioid overuse, other substance abuse, low functional status, potentially unclear pain etiology, and exaggeration of pain level and severity. Scoring is based on a summation of positive endorsements that can range anywhere from 0 to 6. Higher scores indicate possible aberrant use, with a score of 4 serving as a red flag for such risk. In a case-control study, patients with total scores above 3 evidenced an odds ratio of 16.6 (95% confidence interval: 8.3–33; p ≤ 0.001) for opioid abuse, compared with patients with scores below this cutoff [10].

Initial results from Atluri and Sudarshan [10] appear promising, but it is vital to acknowledge that the study was a retrospective case-control study on patients with nonmalignant chronic pain. This measure has not been assessed in the cancer population or those with acute pain and needs to be applied in prospective clinical trials in order to gain further validation.

Chemical Coping Inventory

The Chemical Coping Inventory (CCI) is still currently in development, and its first trial is underway. What differentiates this instrument from other assessments is its intent to capture attitudes and personality traits that could potentially lead to the maladaptive progress toward practical goals, problematic drug use and an overreliance on medication to cope with and manage chronic pain [11].

The CCI anticipates classifying comorbid characteristics with intention of and potential for abuse by a 15-item, 1-factor scale. The CCI assesses somatization, sensation seeking, alexithymia and overcentrality of drug taking. Kirsh et al. [11] have recognized a vast middle ground of chronic pain patients that have a propensity for developing drug use problems that are not necessarily indicative of true addiction. The inventory is designed to separate these patients from those with a classic substance use disorder.

Preliminary progress has been promising, with focus groups of professionals and patients reporting that the items were clear and understandable. The CCI would add a new element to pain treatment planning. It would bridge the gap between internal and external influences with indicative psychological correlates allowing for early integration of psychological treatment and support.

Diagnosis, Intractability, Risk, and Efficacy Score

The Diagnosis, Intractability, Risk and Efficacy (DIRE) score [12] is a clinician-rated scale that predicts both patient compliance and analgesic efficacy of long-term opioid treatment in noncancer pain patients. The scale's title denotes the 4 main categories. The 'risk' category is further divided into 4 subcategories: psychological, chemical health, reliability and social support. Patients with scores above 14 are considered good candidates for opioid treatment, while patients with lower scores have a potential risk for abuse. In a retrospective analysis, Belgrade et al. [12] found that all factors besides 'diagnosis' were significantly related to treatment compliance. It should be noted that though diagnosis is not correlated to compliance, it is included in the measure to rule out patients without conditions associated with moderate or severe pain. In this study, the DIRE score was very successful at predicting patient compliance, with a sensitivity of 94% and a specificity of 87%, as well as at predicting analgesic efficacy, at 81 and 76%, respectively.

Though the results of the study by Belgrade et al. [12] regarding the DIRE score are very appealing, it is important to note that the study was retrospective and scores may have been biased by case history. Additionally, the population was small and included patients with many types of chronic pain. While additional prospective studies must be done to further validate its utility, the DIRE score has great potential for healthcare providers who prefer clinician-based (as opposed to patient-submitted) reports as the DIRE score would help systematize and quantify the clinicians' observations [12].

Opioid Risk Tool

Based on past research, the Opioid Risk Tool (ORT) covers those factors most closely associated with substance abuse. There are 5 'yes' or 'no' items on the dimensions of psychological disease, history of preadolescent sexual abuse, age, and personal and family history of substance abuse [13]. Total ORT scores below 3 indicate a low risk for drug addiction, while scores between 4 and 7 suggest a moderate risk, and total scores above 8 predict a high risk. The total score is achieved by finding the sum of positive endorsements on each of the 5 questions. A score for each positive response is determined specifically by patient gender, and the ORT has demonstrated exceptional discriminatory ability in both men and women (c statistical value of 0.82 and 0.85, respectively). The self-administered ORT can be completed in the waiting area and utilized throughout treatment in order to track or recognize potential abuse.

Due to the brevity and simple scoring of the ORT, there is evident convenience in its use. However, like any self-reported diagnostic tool, it is highly vulnerable to deception. Consequently, there may be a divide among clinicians in terms of preference to use the ORT versus a tool that is longer and more cumbersome, but less susceptible to deception.

Screener and Opioid Assessment for Patients with Pain

The Screener and Opioid Assessment for Patients with Pain-Revised (SOAPP-R) was conceptually devised as a screening tool for assessing abuse potential in patients prior to the initiation of opioid therapy. The SOAPP-R is a 14-item self-report measure that is measured on a 5-point scale ranging from 0 (never) to 4 (very often), with a total score of 8 or greater suggesting a high risk of misuse/abuse [14, 15]. The SOAPP-R has undergone a number of revisions and the relatively low cutoff score of 8 was chosen to potentially account for the patients' underreporting of behaviors.

The SOAPP-R has displayed good psychometric properties, even though the data was correlational and not causal in nature. Also, during the validation of the SOAPP-R, little demographic and medical information was collected, so the baseline risk for the cohort is unknown. Regardless of these concerns, the SOAPP-R could be a clinically valuable screening tool in high-risk pain populations with the continued support of a research program.

Screening Instrument for Substance Abuse Potential

The Screening Instrument for Substance Abuse Potential (SISAP) is a physician-administered, 5-item tool. The SISAP is easy to use and takes only a few minutes for a physician to administer. Following each of the 5 items are two possible directives for the administrator. Based on the response of the patient, the physician will either be advised to stop questions and use caution in prescribing or to proceed to the next question. These 5 questions were developed using data from the National Alcohol and Drug Survey. The 5 questions extracted from the National Alcohol and Drug Survey inquire about the number of drinks on a typical day and in a typical week, use of marijuana in the past year, history of cigarette smoking, and age [16].

A large database of approximately 5,000 pain patients validated this screening tool. When tested, the SISAP illustrated a specificity of 78%, a sensitivity of 91% and an accuracy of 80% for patients who may be at risk of abusing opioids [16]. Notably, the low reported rate of false negatives suggests the SISAP could serve as a quick and simple way to screen substance abuse in a clinical setting.

Despite its initial validation with a notably large cohort of patients, it is unknown why there has not been more testing since the SISAP emerged several years ago. One hypothesis as to the lack of evolution and implementation of the SISAP is that it requires clinicians to ask a collection of specific questions related to alcohol and drug abuse. Nonetheless, its brevity is appealing and additional validation is required to determine the tool's capacity and usefulness in a clinical pain setting.

Screening Tool for Addiction Risk

The Screening Tool for Addiction Risk (STAR) consists of 14 self-administered yes-or-no questions on addiction risk in chronic pain patients. The questions of the STAR cover: cigarette, alcohol and drug use; family or household members with drug or alcohol abuse; visits to pain clinics and emergency rooms, and feelings of depression, anxiety and altered mood. Out of those dimensions listed, individuals responding 'yes' to screening questions related to abusing tobacco products, prior treatment in a drug or alcohol rehabilitation facility, or treatment in another pain clinic were more likely to be patients with existing substance abuse ($p < 0.05$). Analysis suggested that the most significant predictor of addiction was a history of treatment in a drug or alcohol rehabilitation clinic (positive predictive value: 93%; negative predictive value: 5.9%) [17].

Similar to most self-report measures, the STAR has a risk for deception and no correction for lying; however, it has the potential to aid in screening and treatment planning due to its brevity. It has been used with chronic pain patients, but there is a need for larger prospective studies to examine the tool's ability to predict aberrant drug-related behaviors.

Screening Tools for Nonpain Populations

Drug Abuse Problem Assessment for Primary Care

The Drug Abuse Problem Assessment for Primary Care (DAPA-PC) is used to screen adult populations for drug and alcohol abuse problems. As one of few assessments, the DAPA-PC is an Internet-based screening tool. There are two levels to this comprehensive computerized system, which was produced under contract with the National Institute on Drug Abuse [18]. Based on the responses to the health and safety screen, which discretely explores substance abuse through associated components of risk and trauma (i.e. depression and physical/emotional abuse) over the past 5 years, the patients may be asked to also complete the drug and alcohol problem screen, which focuses more directly on drug and alcohol abuse through a series of 12 questions. Patients can complete the entire module privately on a designated computer in the waiting room prior to the first clinic visit. Results are posted immediately to the patient, and if a risk of alcohol or drug abuse exists, motivational messages, advice and additional resources are provided as well. Through this system, the patients' records and useful healthcare-related links can later be accessed by the clinician to assist in the patients' care.

Compared to other assessments, the DAPA-PC is arguably more likely to elicit honest responses due to its completion in privacy. Electronic formatting may provide optimal support to clinics with electronic medical records, and the computer administration and scoring saves time and staffing. The DAPA-PC has great potential for utility in pain clinics, but first requires validation among chronic pain patients.

Drug Abuse Screening Test

The DAST is a unidimensional scale that can be administered in either a self-report or a structured interview format with 'yes' or 'no' responses. Items investigate potential involvement with different classes of drugs including prescribed, over-the-counter and illegal drugs. The quick administration and scoring time, in addition to the low price of the assessment, makes it feasible in a variety of settings, regardless of time and financial challenges [19].

There are many validated versions of the DAST: the original 28-item test, a 20-item test, a 10-item test, and an adolescent-directed test. Psychometrics with all versions are excellent, with options of choosing different cutoff scores to obtain desired results of either sensitivity or specificity. After necessary validation trials have been conducted in pain populations, this measure, particularly the briefer versions, could be useful for pretreatment assessments in pain clinics. However, while this assessment successfully predicts substance abuse, it is unknown whether it specifically predicts aberrant behavior during pain treatment.

Kreek-McHugh-Schluger-Kellogg Scale

Surfacing in 2003, the Kreek-McHugh-Schluger-Kellogg (KMSK) Scale focuses primarily on a patient's time of heaviest use of opioids, cocaine or alcohol. The 8-item tool has separate scales for each substance and assesses the frequency, amount, duration, mode of use and preference of substance for the individual. Analyses of sums on all 3 subscales suggest an impressive ability to indentify dependence (for opioids, a cutoff of 9 offered a positive predictive value of 95%, and a negative predictive value of 100%); however, only the alcohol subscale was able to predict severity of dependence [20].

Kellogg and his colleagues are planning to create similar tests for benzodiazepines (sedatives), barbiturates (sleeping pills) and marijuana. A specific test for pain medication does not appear to be on the horizon. Because the KMSK has failed to quantify drug dependence severity except for alcohol, it does not contribute much to the existing battery of screening measures for pain management clinicians.

Substance Abuse Subtle Screening Inventory

The Substance Abuse Subtle Screening Inventory (SASSI) is an instrument designed as an objective measurement of substance dependence of an individual. The third version of the SASSI (SASSI-3) includes both face-valid items that are direct in delivery on lifetime regularity of specific behaviors related to substance use, as well as subtle true-or-false items that have no apparent relationship to substance abuse.

The SASSI-3 has excellent psychometrics and is very promising. The internal consistency of the SASSI-3 is high, with an α coefficient of 0.93. In a cross-validation comparison of 381 patients with clinical diagnoses based on the DSM-III-R, the SASSI-3 offered an overall accuracy of 97%, a sensitivity of 97% and a specificity of 95%. The positive predictive power measured 99%, and the negative predictive power was 90% [21].

The SASSI-3 can be used in a large variety of clinical settings. It is relevant for the early identification of people who may have substance dependence or susceptibility to one. The SASSI-3 acknowledges relevant symptoms that the individual may not perceive. Deception by the individual is potentially averted due to the design of the inventory. Testing consistency, administration and results of the SASSI make it a valuable tool for a clinical setting.

Two-Item Conjoint Screen

Commonly used in the primary care setting for rapid administration, the Two-Item Conjoint Screen (TICS) aids in the identification of patients with current alcohol or drug problems [22]. The 2-item conjoined questions are scored on a 4-point scale ranging from 0 (never) to 4 (often); however, a response of 'rarely', 'sometimes' or 'often' will be interpreted as a positive reply. This approach allows patients to minimize their responses while still answering in a positive manner. The items on the TICS were conjoined to inquire about alcohol and drug use simultaneously with the intended purpose of encouraging truthful positive endorsements by eliminating fear of legal consequence, particular drug stigmas and other similar side effects. However, this may have an adverse effect on those only using alcohol, for fear that they may be considered drug users as well.

Brown et al. [22] whittled down a 5-item measure to the current 2-item version, reporting that the 3 items eliminated yielded no additional improvement in the detection of substance abuse. Though the TICS has a high negative predictive value of 92.7%, the positive predictive value is only 51.8%. Furthermore, this tool is more sensitive to dependence than abuse, and has a high false-positive rate. Therefore, despite the advantage of its speed, the TICS probably has little relevance to the pain management clinician.

Interview Tools

Addiction Severity Index (ASI)

The Addiction Severity Index (ASI) was developed to function in a host of settings while remaining standardized and reliable [23, 24]. The ASI is noted as one of the most widely used assessments in the USA for treatment planning, as well as for determining substance abuse-related problems and severity. It is administered as a semi-structured interview that addresses 7 dimensions that have been identified as problem areas in individuals abusing substances. The ASI inquires about a patient's medical status, legal status, alcohol use, employment and support, drug use, family/social status and psychiatric status. The clinician asks about the relevance of each factor over the past month, in addition to within the patient's lifetime. The severity rating scales range from 0 (no treatment necessary) to 9 (treatment needed to intervene in life-threatening situation). Though its interview format may be time consuming, the ASI may prove useful in making finer distinctions among patients with problems with drug abuse.

Alcohol and Drug Diagnostic Instrument and Substance Use Disorder Diagnostic Schedule

The Alcohol and Drug Diagnostic Instrument (ADDIS), an adaptation of the Substance Use Disorder Diagnostic Schedule (SUDDS), is a structured interview lasting about 45–60 min designed to allow a diagnosis of substance use dependence in accordance with DSM-III-R criteria [25]. The ADDIS has been found to be useful in a number of clinical settings to assess the prevalence of abuse and dependency.

Jonasson et al. [25] conducted a study in Sweden administering the ADDIS to 243 orthopedic and chronic pain patients. According to DSM-III-R standards, 33% had some form of substance abuse disorder, two thirds of which were analgesic abuse/dependence. Although when applying the criteria of the DSM-IV, the prevalence was lower (26%, with a similar distribution of analgesic disorders), substance abuse/dependence was still pervasive. Even though the structured interview of the ADDIS/SUDDS may be time consuming, they are both still useful instruments in assessing dependence or abuse in chronic pain patients.

Documentation

Pain Assessment and Documentation Tool

It is essential that physicians assess patients before selecting a pain management plan and continue to monitor after its initiation. During follow-up, it is also essential that physicians actively pay attention to a patient's analgesia, activities of daily living, adverse effects and other aberrant drug-related behaviors. These 4 domains are referred to as the '4 As'. When considering whether a patient should maintain the chosen treatment plan, the most significant 'A' domain to reference would be the last, i.e. aberrant drug-taking behaviors. This broad domain is composed of a wide range of abnormal behaviors related to drug use [26].

The Pain Assessment and Documentation Tool (PADT) was created by Passik and colleagues to implement consistent documentation of the progress of the 4 As. The 2-sided chart of the PADT provides a focus on key outcomes and pain management in therapy over the course of time. The overall objective was to design a simple charting device that had was fast to complete and was an easy addition to a patient's medical record. In order to ensure the PADT met the objective of the developers, controlled field tests of the PADT allowed for clinicians to refine and revise the chart accordingly. Therefore, the PADT has demonstrated its ability to be pragmatic and intuitive, and to have seamless integration into any clinical situation. The absence of strict scoring criteria for the PADT charting tool distinguishes the device from other assessment and documentation tools. Evidence from previous trials suggests that abuse and possible addiction can be predicted over a 6-month period if 4 or more aberrant behaviors are shown.

Discussion

Though fairly comprehensive, this list is by no means exhaustive or inclusive of all potentially useful assessment tools for managing pain and predicting substance abuse in chronic pain patients. It should be noted that no prospectively defined criteria assessing the strengths of the study designs were employed in creating this list. In addition, the selection of measures may have been subjectively biased by the authors' experience.

The measures described above vary in administration style, psychometrics and intended applications. Some of them, such as the SOAPP, DIRE and ORT, are targeted at assessing the potential for substance abuse prior to treatment. Once a patient has begun taking opioids, certain measures (TICS, KMSK Scale, DAST, DAPA-PC and SASSI) successfully assess current alcohol and/or drug abuse. Other tools, like the ADDIS/SUDDS, provide structure for diagnosis of a substance use disorder.

Conclusion

Addiction to pain medications is a growing health concern in the USA. Opioids are a useful treatment option in chronic pain and cancer patients, yet clinicians cannot ignore the potential risk for these drugs to be misused and abused. The medical community should utilize screening tools prior to and throughout pain treatment to best serve both the clinician and the patient. Although some of these measures still need to be further tested, this list should serve as a good first step toward optimal pain management.

References

1 Argoff CE: The coexistence of neuropathic pain, sleep, and psychiatric disorders: a novel treatment approach. Clin J Pain 2007;23:15–22.

2 Cicero TJ, Inciardi JA, Muñoz A: Trends in abuse of Oxycontin and other opioid analgesics in the United States: 2002–2004. J Pain 2005;6:662–672.

3 Lipman AG: Does the DEA truly seek balance in pain medicine? A chronology of confusion that impedes good patient care. J Pain Palliat Care Pharmacother 2005;19:7–9.

4 Volkow ND: Scientific research on prescription drug abuse, before the Subcommittee on Crime and Drugs, Committee on the Judiciary and the Caucus on International Narcotics Control United States Senate. 2008. http://www.drugabuse.gov/Testimony/3-12–08Testimony.html (accessed May 10, 2008).

5 NSDUH Report: Patterns and trends in nonmedical prescription pain reliever use: 2002 to 2005. Rockville, Substance Abuse and Mental Health Services Administration, 2007.

6 Results from the 2005 National Survey on Drug Use and Health: national findings. 2006. http://www.oas.samhsa.gov/NSDUH/2k5NSDUH/2k5results.htm (accessed May 10, 2008).

7 Cleeland CS, Ryan KM: Pain assessment: global use of the Brief Pain Inventory. Ann Acad Med Singapore 1994;23:129–138.

8 Kroenke K, Spitzer RL, Williams JB: The PHQ-9: validity of a brief depression severity measure. J Gen Intern Med 2001;16:606–613.

9 Stratford PW, Binkley J, Solomon P, Finch E, Gill C, Moreland J: Defining the minimum level of detectable change for the Roland-Morris questionnaire. Phys Ther 1996;76:359–365, discussion 366–368.

10 Atluri SL, Sudarshan G: Development of a screening tool to detect the risk of inappropriate prescription opioid use in patients with chronic pain. Pain Physician 2004;7:333–338.

11 Kirsh K, Jass C, Bennett DS, Hagen JE, Passik SD: Initial development of a survey tool to detect issues of chemical coping in chronic pain patients. Palliat Support Care 2007;5:219–226.

12 Belgrade MJ, Schamber CD, Lindgren BR: The DIRE score: predicting outcomes of opioid prescribing for chronic pain. J Pain 2006;7:671–681.

13 Webster LR, Webster RM: Predicting aberrant behaviors in opioid-treated patients: preliminary validation of the Opioid Risk Tool. Pain Med 2005;6:432–442.

14 Butler SF, Budman SH, Fernandez K, Jamison RN: Validation of a screener and opioid assessment measure for patients with chronic pain. Pain 2004;112:65–75.

15 Akbik H, Butler SF, Budman SH, Fernandez K, Katz NP, Jamison RN: Validation and clinical application of the Screener and Opioid Assessment for Patients with Pain (SOAPP). J Pain Symptom Manage 2006;32:287–293.

16 Coambs R, Jarry JL, Santhiapillai AC, Abrahamsohn RV, et al: The SISAP: a new screening instrument for identifying potential opioid abusers in the management of chronic nonmalignant pain within general medical practice. Pain Res Manag 1996;1:155–162.

17 Passik SD, Kirsh KL, Casper D: Addiction-related assessment tools and pain management: instruments for screening, treatment planning, and monitoring compliance. Pain Med 2008;9:S145–S166.

18 Nemes S, Rao PA, Zeiler C, Munly K, Holtz KD, Hoffman J: Computerized screening of substance abuse problems in a primary care setting: older vs younger adults. Am J Drug Alcohol Abuse 2004;30:627–642.

19 Yudko E, Lozhkina O, Fouts A: A comprehensive review of the psychometric properties of the Drug Abuse Screening Test. J Subst Abuse Treat 2007;32:189–198.

20 Kellogg SH, McHugh PF, Bell K, Schluger JH, Schluger RP, LaForge KS, Ho A, Kreek MJ: The Kreek-McHugh-Schluger-Kellogg scale: a new, rapid method for quantifying substance abuse and its possible applications. Drug Alcohol Depend 2003;69:137–150.

21 Lazowski LE, Miller FG, Boye MW, Miller GA: Efficacy of the Substance Abuse Subtle Screening Inventory-3 (SASSI-3) in identifying substance dependence disorders in clinical settings. J Pers Assess 1998;71:114–128.

22 Brown RL, Leonard T, Saunders LA, Papasouliotis O: A two-item conjoint screen for alcohol and other drug problems. J Am Board Fam Pract 2001;14:95–106.

23 Cacciola JS, Alterman AI, O'Brien CP, McLellan AT: The Addiction Severity Index in clinical efficacy trials of medications for cocaine dependence. NIDA Res Monogr 1997;175:182–191.

24 McLellan AT, Luborsky L, Woody GE, O'Brien CP: An improved diagnostic evaluation instrument for substance abuse patients: the Addiction Severity Index. J Nerv Ment Dis 1980;168:26–33.

25 Jonasson U, Jonasson B, Wickström L, Andersson E, Saldeen T: Analgesic use disorders among orthopedic and chronic pain patients at a rehabilitation clinic. Subst Use Misuse 1998;33:1375–1385.

26 Passik SD, Weinreb HJ: Managing chronic nonmalignant pain: overcoming obstacles to the use of opioids. Adv Ther 2000;17:70–83.

Steven D. Passik, PhD
Department of Psychiatry and Behavioral Sciences, Memorial Sloan-Kettering Cancer Center
641 Lexington Avenue, 7th Floor
New York, NY 10022 (USA)
Tel. +1 646 888 0022, E-Mail passiks@mskcc.org

Clark MR, Treisman GJ (eds): Chronic Pain and Addiction.
Adv Psychosom Med. Basel, Karger, 2011, vol 30, pp 125–138

Cannabinoids for Pain Management

Adam Thaler[a] · Anita Gupta[a] · Steven P. Cohen[b,c]

[a]Pain Management Division, Department of Anesthesiology, University of Pennsylvania School of Medicine, Philadelphia, Pa., [b]Pain Management Division, Department of Anesthesiology and Critical Care Medicine, Johns Hopkins School of Medicine, Baltimore, Md., and [c]Department of Surgery, Walter Reed Army Medical Center, Washington, D.C., USA

Abstract

Cannabinoids have been used for thousands of years to provide relief from suffering, but only recently have they been critically evaluated in clinical trials. This review provides an in-depth examination of the evidence supporting cannabinoids in various pain states, along with an overview of potential adverse effects. In summary, there is strong evidence for a moderate analgesic effect in peripheral neuropathic and central pain conditions, and conflicting evidence for their use in nociceptive pain. For spasticity, most controlled studies demonstrate significant improvement. Adverse effects are not uncommon with cannabinoids, though most are not serious and self-limiting. In view of the limited effect size and low but not inconsequential risk of serious adverse events, cannabinoids should be employed as analgesics only when safer and more effective medication trials have failed, or as part of a multimodal treatment regimen.

Copyright © 2011 S. Karger AG, Basel

History

Cannabis preparations have been used as medicinal agents for thousands of years. Use of the plant was first described in a medical context by the Chinese emperor Shen Nung in 2700 BCE to treat beriberi, gout, malaria, rheumatism and numerous other conditions [1]. Cannabis was cultivated in Europe and Asia as a fiber plant and ultimately became a central nonconsumable crop in colonial and postrevolutionary America. George Washington is believed to have smoked hemp to relieve tooth pain. In 1799, Napoleon Bonaparte's army returned to France from an unsuccessful Egyptian campaign with soldiers who carried extensive knowledge of the plant. Napoleon's scientists were amongst the first Western Europeans to study cannabinoid effects methodically; two of them, Silvestre de Sacy and P.C. Rouyer, published papers on cannabinoids touching off a new round of medical inquiry [1].

Mechanism of Action of Cannabinoids

Δ^9-Tetrahydrocannabinol (THC) is the main source of the pharmacological effects of cannabinoids. However, its acidic metabolite THC-COOH and several other analogues and constituents are also promising candidates for therapeutic uses [2]. The active ingredient is thought to exert most of its effects via cannabinoid CB_1 receptors located on presynaptic nerve terminals in the brain and peripheral tissues. CB_1 activity is mediated by G proteins via several signal transduction pathways. G proteins directly inhibit N- and P/Q-type, voltage-dependent calcium channels and sodium channels, and indirectly inhibit A-type calcium channels via inhibition of adenylate cyclase. Δ^9-THC binding and G protein activation also activate inwardly rectifying potassium channels and the mitogen-activated protein kinase signaling pathway [3]. In addition, there is increasing evidence for nonreceptor-mediated antinociceptive mechanisms.

Synthetic versus Natural Cannabinoids

Naturally occurring cannabinoids are biosynthetically related, terpene-phenolic compounds produced by the plant *Cannabis sativa* L. Natural and synthetic cannabinoids have been extensively studied since the discovery that the psychotropic effects of cannabinoids are mainly due to Δ^9-THC. The FDA approval of dronabinol in 1985 as an antiemetic in cancer patients receiving chemotherapy, and later as an appetite stimulant in AIDS patients, has further intensified research endeavors [4].

Synthetic compounds can be classified as either classical or nonclassical formulations. Classical cannabinoids retain their natural cannabinoid ring structure and oxygen atom. Nabilone, a ketocannabinoid, is the only classical synthetic compound currently in use. It recently received FDA approval as a treatment for nausea and vomiting associated with chemotherapy [1]. Nonclassical cannabinoids exhibit either a rearrangement or deletion of the prototypical pyran B ring of classical cannabinoids. Hybrid cannabinoids combine the pharmacophoric features of classical and nonclassical cannabinoids.

Pharmacokinetics and Pharmacodynamics of Cannabinoids

Increasing interest in the medicinal use of cannabinoid medications necessitates an understanding of pharmacokinetics and disposition into biological tissues. A drug's pharmacokinetics determines the onset, magnitude and duration of its pharmacodynamic effects. Natural cannabinoid products are usually inhaled or taken orally; alternative routes have only been sporadically used and are of little clinical relevance. The pharmacokinetics of THC vary as a function of its route of administration. Because of its high lipid solubility, topical administration is possible in such locations as the eye or nasal mucosa, though this tends to be irritating and poorly tolerated. However, newer vehicles that permit lipid-soluble materials to be applied in aqueous solution may someday change this. THC can also be converted to a hemisuccinate and administered as a rectal suppository, which results in much higher bioavailability than with oral administration. In addition, rectal absorption delivers the drug directly into the systemic circulation, thus avoiding the first-pass metabolism. Pulmonary assimilation of inhaled THC results in a maximum plasma concentration within minutes, achieving a peak effect after 15–30 min, and dissipates within 2–3 h. Oral administration results in a slow and variable absorption, with a bioavailability of 10–20%. Following oral ingestion, psychotropic effects occur in 30–90 min, reach their maximum effect after 2–3 h and can last between 4 and 12 h depending on the dose [2]. Although there is first-pass metabolism in the liver, the major metabolite, 11-hydroxy-THC, is at least as potent as THC itself. Hence, this does not result in decreased efficacy [5].

THC and its analogues have shown significant therapeutic benefits in the relief of nausea and vomiting, and in the stimulation of appetite in patients with wasting syndrome. Recent evidence also demonstrates modest analgesic and antispasticity effects. The ability of cannabinoids to reduce intraocular pressure in glaucoma, and to dilate bronchi in asthma, is neither strong enough nor of sufficient duration or reliability to justify their use for these conditions at present. However, the anticonvulsant effects of cannabinoids are sufficiently promising to warrant further clinical investigation [2, 5].

There are two main cannabinoid receptors in the human body. CB_1 receptors are found in high concentrations in the basal ganglia, limbic system, hypothalamus, dorsal horn and cerebellum, and in lower concentrations in the reproductive system. The CB_1 receptor is responsible for euphoric and anticonvulsive effects. The CB_2 receptor is found almost exclusively in the immune and hematopoietic systems. In the nervous system, it is predominantly expressed on peripheral nerve terminals, though a subpopulation has been described on microglia in human cerebellum. This receptor is responsible for the anti-inflammatory and immunosuppressive actions of cannabinoids [2, 5].

Evidence of Efficacy

Nociceptive Pain
Experimental and clinical studies evaluating the effects of cannabinoids on nociceptive pain have been decidedly mixed (table 1). Wallace et al. [6] found a modest analgesic effect for a medium dose of smoked cannabis on capsaicin-induced pain, but at higher doses an increase in pain was noted. In contrast, Kraft et al. [7] found no significant analgesic effects for oral Δ^9-THC on capsaicin- and heat-induced pain thresholds. However, the ingestion of THC lowered electrical pain thresholds

Table 1. Randomized controlled studies evaluating cannabinoids for nociceptive pain

Study	Study design	Patients	Results
Beaulieu [11]	Randomized, double-blind, placebo-controlled, parallel group with active comparator	41 patients undergoing gynecological (46%), orthopedic (44%) or other treatment	Nabilone 1 mg = placebo > nabilone 2 mg over 24 h
Blake et al. [15]	Randomized, double-blind, parallel group	58 patients with rheumatoid arthritis	Oromucosal THC: cannabidiol > placebo over 5 weeks
Buggy et al. [10]	Randomized, double-blind, placebo-controlled	40 women undergoing elective abdominal hysterectomy	Δ^9-THC no different from placebo for 24 h
Noyes Jr. et al. [38]	Randomized, double-blind, placebo-controlled	36 patients with cancer	THC > placebo
Wallace et al. [6]	Randomized, double-blind, placebo-controlled, crossover	15 healthy patients	Medium dose (4% Δ^9-THC) smoked cannabis > placebo and low dose (2%) > high dose (8%) in pain decrease over 45 min
Kraft et al. [7]	Randomized, double-blind, placebo-controlled	18 healthy females	Cannabis < placebo over 8 h
Redmond et al. [8]	Randomized, double-blind, placebo-controlled, crossover	17 patients (10 women, 7 men)	Nabilone highest strength (1 mg) > placebo after 2 h only for women

compared to baseline and placebo. In a study examining the effects of the synthetic cannabinoid nabilone on experimental heat pain, Redmond et al. [8] found no evidence for antinociception in the general study population. However, subgroup analysis determined that higher doses (1 mg) of nabilone significantly reduced temporal summation in women. With respect to the ability of cannabinoids to attenuate postoperative pain, some uncontrolled studies have yielded auspicious results [9], whereas controlled studies have failed to show any benefit [10, 11]. Preclinical studies have demonstrated that cannabinoids may have anti-inflammatory effects, and reduce joint injury, in arthritis [12–14]. In a randomized, double-blind, placebo-controlled study conducted on 58 patients with rheumatoid arthritis, Blake et al. [15] found that

Table 2. Randomized controlled studies evaluating cannabinoids for neuropathic pain

Study	Study design	Patients	Results
Ellis et al. [17]	Phase II, randomized, double-blind, placebo-controlled, crossover	28 patients with HIV-associated distal sensory-predominant polyneuropathy	Smoked cannabis > placebo in pain reduction over 5 days
Wilsey et al. [39]	Randomized, placebo-controlled, crossover	38 patients with central/peripheral neuropathic pain	Smoked cannabis > placebo over 3 weeks
Frank et al. [40]	Randomized, crossover, double-blind	96 patients with neuropathic pain	Dihydrocodeine > synthetic cannabinoid nabilone over 6 weeks
Nurmikko et al. [16]	Randomized, double-blind, placebo-controlled	125 patients with neuropathic pain and allodynia	Oromucosal THC: cannabidiol > placebo over 5 weeks; maintained for 52 weeks in open-label extension
Abrams et al. [18]	Prospective, randomized, placebo-controlled	50 patients with painful HIV-associated sensory neuropathy	Smoked cannabis > placebo over 5 days
Notcutt et al. [41]	Randomized, double-blind, placebo-controlled, crossover	34 'N of 1' studies in patients with chronic, mostly neuropathic pain	Sublingual spray THC and cannabidiol > placebo over 12 weeks
Karst et al. [42]	Randomized, double-blind, placebo-controlled, crossover	21 patients with recalcitrant neuropathic pain and hyperalgesia	$1',1'$-Dimethylheptyl-Δ^8-tetrahydrocannabinol-11-oic acid (CT-3) > placebo for two 7-day treatment periods

oromucosal Sativex, a natural cannabinoid, resulted in significant improvements in pain relief, functional capacity and sleep compared to placebo.

Peripheral Neuropathic Pain

Studies evaluating cannabinoids have demonstrated their efficacy in treating neuropathic pain [16, 17] (table 2). Nurmikko et al. [16] performed a double-blind, placebo-controlled, parallel study evaluating oromucosal Sativex in 125 patients with peripheral neuropathic pain. By the 5-week follow-up, the treatment group had experienced significant improvement in pain scores, allodynia, functional capacity and sleep compared to the control group. The benefit was maintained without dose escalation or toxicity for 52 weeks in an open-label extension. In a phase II, double-blind, placebo-controlled crossover trial, Ellis et al. [17] assessed the impact of smoked cannabinoid on neuropathic pain in HIV-related neuropathy (primarily distal sensory-predominant polyneuropathy). The treatment group received between 1 and 8% Δ^9-THC titrated to effect 4 times daily for 5 consecutive days. For the 28 patients who completed the study, pain relief was significantly greater in the treatment group, with 46% achieving at least 30% pain relief with cannabinoids compared to 18% with placebo. Similar beneficial effects on HIV-related neuropathy have been reported in other controlled studies [18]. In addition to pain relief, other beneficial effects of cannabinoids in HIV infection include increased food intake and mood improvement [19].

Central Pain

Central pain conditions such as those associated with multiple sclerosis (MS), spinal cord injury and limb amputation have been shown to benefit from treatment with cannabinoids (table 3). Reviews and meta-analyses have concluded there is moderate evidence to support the use of various cannabinoids to treat the central dysesthetic pain associated with MS [20–22]. However, these drugs are generally not recommended as first-line treatments for a variety of reasons including the side effect profile, modest effect size and short follow-up periods in placebo-controlled studies [23, 24]. In addition, not all randomized controlled trials have demonstrated significant pain improvement in MS subjects with cannabinoid treatment [25].

The evidence supporting cannabinoids in other central pain states is less robust. Wade et al. [26] conducted a series of double-blind, placebo-controlled, single-patient crossover studies on 24 patients with central pain secondary to MS (n = 18), spinal cord injury (n = 4), brachial plexopathy and phantom limb pain (n = 2). Over the 2-week treatment periods, the authors found Δ^9-THC and cannabidiol provided superior analgesia compared to placebo. In another single-patient, placebo-controlled crossover study, Maurer et al. [27] found analgesic effects for both Δ^9-THC and codeine, but not for placebo.

Spasticity

Animal models have demonstrated that both endogenous and exogenous cannabinoids, acting via cannabinoid receptors with an ensuing inhibition of spinal polysynaptic reflexes, may reduce spasticity and tremors [28] (table 4). Numerous randomized controlled studies have evaluated the efficacy of cannabinoids in spasticity due to a wide array of disease states, with most demonstrating significant benefit. For MS, most [29–33] but not all [34] controlled studies have demonstrated reduced spasticity with cannabinoids. Still other studies have demonstrated mixed results. Wissel et al. [35] found the synthetic cannabinoid nabilone to be

Table 3. Randomized controlled studies evaluating cannabinoids for central pain

Study	Study design	Patients	Results
Rog et al. [23]	Randomized, double-blind, placebo-controlled	66 patients with MS	Oromucosal THC/cannabidiol > placebo over 4 weeks
Wade et al. [25]	Randomized, double-blind, placebo-controlled, parallel group	160 outpatients with MS	Oromucosal spray THC/cannabidiol > placebo over 6 weeks
Berman et al. [43]	Randomized, double-blind, placebo-controlled, 3-period, crossover	48 patients with brachial plexopathy	Two cannabis extracts > placebo, but not clinically significant for three 2-week treatment periods
Svendsen et al. [24]	Randomized, double-blind, placebo-controlled, crossover	24 patients with MS	Dronabinol > placebo over 3 weeks
Wade et al. [26]	Randomized, double-blind, placebo-controlled, single-patient, crossover	24 patients with MS, spinal cord injury, brachial plexus damage and limb amputation due to neurofibromatosis	Sublingual spray cannabidiol/THC > placebo over 2 weeks

superior to placebo in reducing spasticity-related pain, but not spasticity, motor function or functional capacity. In another placebo-controlled crossover study, Vaney et al. [36] found a significant reduction in MS-related spasticity in patients who were titrated to ≥90% of the 30 mg/day target dose of THC (per-protocol analysis), but not in the overall 50-patient cohort (intention-to-treat analysis). For spasticity secondary to spinal cord injury, the evidence in support of cannabinoids is more limited. Hagenbach et al. [37] conducted a three-phase open-label study on 25 patients, evaluating oral and rectal THC for spinal cord injury-related spasticity, with a small (n = 13) placebo-controlled phase comparing oral Δ^9-THC with a control group. The authors found significant improvements in both orally and suppository-treated patients who received daily doses of ≥15 mg, with a significant difference noted between the drug and control treatments in the 7 subjects treated with oral THC in phase I and placebo in phase III. In one of the earliest placebo-controlled studies, Petro and Ellenberger Jr. [29] found a significant reduction in spasticity secondary to multiple etiologies in 9 patients following oral THC but not placebo treatment.

Table 4. Randomized controlled studies evaluating cannabinoids for spasticity

Study	Study design	Patients	Results
Collin et al. [31]	Randomized, double-blind, placebo-controlled	189 subjects with MS and spasticity	Oromucosal Δ^9-THC > placebo over 6 weeks
Hagenbach et al. [37]	3-phase, with third phase randomized, double-blind, placebo-controlled	25 patients with spinal cord injury	15–20 mg oral Δ^9-THC + rectal THC hemisuccinate > placebo over 6 weeks
Wissel et al. [35]	Double-blind, placebo-controlled, crossover	11 subjects with MS	Oral nabilone (1 mg) > placebo in decreasing pain for 4 weeks
Vaney et al. [36]	Prospective, randomized, double-blind, placebo-controlled, crossover	57 patients with MS	THC/cannabidiol (2.5 mg/0.9 mg) > placebo over 2 weeks
Zajicek et al. [33]	Multicenter, randomized, placebo-controlled	667 patients with MS	Oral cannabinoid extract and Δ^9-THC > placebo over 15 weeks
Wade et al. [32]	Placebo-controlled, 10-week	137 MS patients with recalcitrant symptoms	Oromucosal cannabis-based medicine (Sativex) > placebo over 10 weeks
Zajicek et al. [56]	Randomized, placebo-controlled	630 patients with stable MS	Oral cannabis extract and Δ^9-THC slightly > placebo over 15 weeks
Killestein et al. [34]	Randomized, double-blind, placebo-controlled, 2-fold crossover	16 patients with MS and severe spasticity	Neither Δ^9-THC, cannabis plant extract nor placebo decreased spasticity for 4 weeks
Ungerleider et al. [30]	Randomized, double-blind, placebo-controlled, crossover	13 patients with MS	THC > placebo in decreasing spasticity per patient for 5 days
Petro and Ellenberger Jr. [29]	Double-blind, placebo-controlled	9 patients with spasticity related to MS	THC > placebo in reducing spasticity

Adverse Effects

Cannabis and its derivatives are associated with euphoria and relaxation, perceptual alterations, time distortion and the intensification of ordinary sensory experiences. The most common unpleasant side effects of occasional cannabinoid use are anxiety

Table 5. Summary of adverse effects of cannabinoids

Organ system	Acute effects	Chronic effects	Possible effects
Respiratory	Bronchodilation; increased forced expiratory volume	Chronic bronchitis; increased risk for respiratory complications; histopathological changes that may be precursors to cancer	Increased risk of lung cancer for inhaled cannabis
Neurological	Impaired attention, memory and psychomotor performance	Possible long-term impairment of attention span and memory	Endocannabinoid system may play a protective or causative role in Alzheimer's disease
Psychiatric	Increased risk of psychotic symptoms in patients genetically predisposed	Physical and psychological dependence; impaired motivation, memory and attention	Impaired educational attainment in adolescents and underachievement in occupations requiring high-level cognitive skills; increased risk of schizophrenia and mood disorders
Gastrointestinal	Delayed gastric emptying; reduced gastric volume; inhibits peristalsis; increased appetite; antiemesis	None	Increased risk of gastrointestinal malignancies
Immunological	Exacerbation of existing allergies	Alveolar macrophage abnormalities; high doses decrease resistance to infection	Immunological tolerance with chronic use; leukemia among offspring exposed in utero

and panic reactions. Cannabinoids also possess cardiovascular effects. Smoking or ingesting THC increases the heart rate by 20–50%, an effect that can last up to 3 h. Blood pressure increases when sitting, but decreases while standing following cannabinoid intake [44]. For a summary of adverse effects of cannabinoids see table 5.

In a systematic review evaluating the adverse effects of cannabinoid-based medicines in 31 studies, Wang et al. [45] found that 97% of adverse events reported in clinical cannabinoid studies were not serious; dizziness was the most common side effect, occurring in 16% of subjects. Although the rate of nonserious adverse events was higher among participants receiving any type of medical cannabinoid than among those allocated to control treatments, significant differences were noted between various preparations. Among individuals receiving oromucosal Δ^9-THC-cannabidiol (rate ratio: 1.88) or oral Δ^9-THC (rate ratio: 2.18), higher rates of nonserious adverse events were reported, while there was no significant difference in studies evaluating oral Δ^9-THC-cannabidiol preparations [45].

In contrast, the rates of serious adverse events were not statistically different between the two groups (rate ratio: 1.04; 95% confidence interval: 0.78–1.39) [45]. However, clear trends were observed, whereby cannabinoid exposure was associated with a higher likelihood of several major side effects. Thirteen percent of patients experienced a relapse in MS. Seventeen percent of subjects exposed to cannabinoids experienced a serious respiratory event (e.g. pneumonia) versus 12% of control patients. For psychiatric side effects (7 vs. 2%) and neoplasm progression (9 vs. 3%), higher rates were also noted for cannabinoid-exposed subjects. In subjects allocated to cannabinoid treatment, the death rates were 3.4 per 100 person-years, compared to 1.3 per 100 person-years in control patients. However, the higher mortality rate was mainly attributable to one study evaluating the effects of Δ^9-THC on cancer-related wasting syndrome [45].

These findings generally support conclusions by the Institute of Medicine that the short-tem use of cannabinoids for medicinal purposes is associated with an acceptable safety profile [46]. But whereas this provides reassurance for clinicians prescribing cannabinoids for short-term symptom palliation, it provides little information on the long-term sequelae of cannabinoid use for chronic disorders [47, 48]. The consequences of most concern to clinicians are psychological dependence, exacerbation of cardiovascular disease, precipitation of psychotic disorders, and cancer. The smoke associated with cannabinoid use may be carcinogenic and has been identified as mutagenic in vitro and in vivo. Cannabinoids weaken cell-mediated and humoral immunity in preclinical studies, decreasing resistance to infection. Noncannabinoid substances in cannabinoid-based cigarettes can also impair alveolar macrophages [44]. Chronic heavy cannabinoid smoking is associated with an increased incidence of bronchitis. In a meta-analysis by Tetrault et al. [49] examining the respiratory effects of marijuana smoking, the authors found strong evidence for short-term bronchodilation and increased forced expiratory volume. No consistent correlation was found between cannabinoid smoking and long-term lung complications, though a majority of studies found a decreased forced expiratory volume/forced vital capacity ratio (an indicator of obstructive lung disease). All 14 studies found an association between chronic marijuana smoking and respiratory complications, with the three most frequent being wheeze, increased sputum production and chronic cough.

Chronic administration of high doses of THC to animals lowers testosterone secretion, impairs sperm production, motility and viability, and disrupts the ovulatory cycle. Whether cannabinoid smoking has these effects in human beings is uncertain because the published evidence is scant and inconsistent. Evidence does suggest that

Thaler · Gupta · Cohen

in utero exposure to cannabinoids can have deleterious behavioral and developmental effects after birth. Even up to 9 years of age, children exposed to cannabinoids in utero can experience deficits in sustained attention, memory and higher cognitive functioning [44]. There is less robust evidence that heavy marijuana use can impede family functioning, reduce psychological well-being and increase criminal behavior. Large doses of THC can produce confusion, amnesia, delusions, hallucinations, anxiety and agitation. In susceptible individuals, cannabinoid abuse can also be an independent risk factor for schizophrenia and psychosis through a variety of mechanisms including an effect on neurodevelopment during adolescence, and dysregulation of the endocannabinoid system [50, 51].

Profound behavioral tolerance can develop in predisposed individuals, and there is a growing body of evidence for physical dependence manifesting as withdrawal symptoms upon cessation in heavy users [52, 53]. However, much of the literature on psychological dependence relies on cohort studies involving recreational users who began using cannabinoids in adolescence. In industrialized countries, cannabinoid dependence is the most common form of illicit drug dependence. Between 7 and 10% of cannabinoid users may develop dependence, with early onset and larger quantity of use both predicting future dependence [44, 53]. There are some reports of an association between dependence and genetic variations in the cannabinoid receptor 1 gene, but to date this evidence has been weak and inconsistent [54, 55].

Conclusions

In summary, controlled studies clearly demonstrate analgesic effects for cannabinoids, though the potential benefits are limited by the narrow therapeutic index and the small effect size. For peripheral and central neuropathic pain states, there is compelling evidence supporting cannabinoids, whereas the evidence for nociceptive pain is conflicting. Aside from regulatory issues, the main drawback to cannabinoid therapy seems to be adverse effects, which to some extent depend on the type and route of administration. Similar to other agents used for neuropathic pain, the most common side effects tend to be neurological. More research is needed to determine the long-term effects of cannabinoid use, to refine selection criteria and to develop compounds with more favorable side effect profiles.

References

1 Geller T: Cannabinoids: a secret history. Chemical Heritage Newsmagazine 2007;25.
2 Grotenhermen F: Pharmacokinetics and pharmacodynamics of cannabinoids. Clin Pharmacokinet 2003;42:327–360.
3 Yamamoto T, Takada K: Role of cannabinoid receptor in the brain as it relates to drug reward. Jpn J Pharmacol 2000;84:229–236.

4 Galal A, Slade D, Gul W, El-Alfy AT, Ferreira D, Elsohly MA: Naturally occurring and related synthetic cannabinoids and their potential therapeutic applications. Recent Pat CNS Drug Discov 2009;4: 112–136.

5 Huestis MA: Pharmacokinetics and metabolism of the plant cannabinoids, Δ^9-tetrahydrocannabinol, cannabidiol and cannabinol. Handb Exp Pharmacol 2005;168:657–690.

6 Wallace M, Schulteis G, Atkinson J, Wolfson T, Lazzaretto D, Bentley H, Gouaux B, Abramson I: Dose-dependent effects of smoked cannabis on capsaicin-induced pain and hyperalgesia in healthy volunteers. Anesthesiology 2007;107: 785–796.

7 Kraft B, Frickey N, Kaufmann R, Reif M, Frey R, Gustorff B, Kress HG: Lack of analgesia by oral standardized cannabis extract on acute inflammatory pain and hyperalgesia in volunteers. Anesthesiology 2008;109:101–110.

8 Redmond W, Goffaux P, Potvin S, Marchand S: Analgesic and antihyperanalgesic effects of nabilone on experimental heat pain. Curr Med Res Opin 2008;24:1017–1024.

9 Holdcroft A, Maze M, Doré C, Tebbs S, Thompson S: A multicenter dose-escalation study of the analgesic and adverse effects of an oral cannabis extract (Cannador) for postoperative pain management. Anesthesiology 2006;104:1040–1046.

10 Buggy D, Toogood L, Maric S, Sharpe P, Lambert DG, Rowbotham DJ: Lack of analgesic efficacy of oral Δ^9-tetrahdrocannabinol in postoperative pain. Pain 2003;106:169–172.

11 Beaulieu P: Effects of nabilone, a synthetic cannabinoid, on postoperative pain. Can J Anaesth 2006;53: 769–775.

12 Selvi E, Lorenzini S, Garcia-Gonzalez E, Maggio R, Lazzerini PE, Capecchi PL, Balistreri E, Spreafico A, Niccolini S, Pompella G, Natale MR, Guideri F, Laghi Pasini F, Galeazzi M, Marcolongo R: Inhibitory effect of synthetic cannabinoids on cytokine production in rheumatoid fibroblast-like synoviocytes. Clin Exp Rheumatol 2008;26: 574–581.

13 Stebulis J, Johnson D, Rossetti R, Burstein SH, Zurier RB: Ajulemic acid, a synthetic cannabinoid acid, induces an antiinflammatory profile of eicosanoids in human synovial cells. Life Sci 2008;83: 666–670.

14 Parker J, Atez F, Rossetti RG, Skulas A, Patel R, Zurier RB: Suppression of human macrophage interleukin-6 by a nonpsychoactive cannabinoid acid. Rheumatol Int 2008;28:631–635.

15 Blake D, Robson P, Ho M, Jubb RW, McCabe CS: Preliminary assessment of the efficacy, tolerability and safety of a cannabis-based medicine (Sativex) in the treatment of pain caused by rheumatoid arthritis. Rheumatology (Oxford) 2006;45:50–52.

16 Nurmikko T, Serpell M, Hoggart B, Toomey PJ, Morlion BJ, Haines D: Sativex successfully treats neuropathic pain characterised by allodynia: a randomised, double-blind, placebo-controlled clinical trial. Pain 2007;133:210–220.

17 Ellis R, Toperoff W, Vaida F, van den Brande G, Gonzales J, Gouaux B, Bentley H, Atkinson JH: Smoked medicinal cannabis for neuropathic pain in HIV: a randomized, crossover clinical trial. Neuropsychopharmacology 2009;34:672–680.

18 Abrams D, Jay C, Shade S, Vizoso H, Reda H, Press S, Kelly ME, Rowbotham MC, Petersen KL: Cannabis in painful HIV-associated sensory neuropathy. Neurology 2007;68:515–521.

19 Haney M, Rabkin J, Gunderson E, Foltin R: Dronabinol and marijuana in HIV+ marijuana smokers: acute effects on caloric intake and mood. Psychopharmacology 2005;181:170–178.

20 Finnerup N, Jensen O, Sindrup S: An evidence-based algorithm for the treatment of neuropathic pain. MedGenMed 2007;9:36.

21 Hosking R, Zajicek J: Therapeutic potential of cannabis in pain medicine. Br J Anaesth 2008;101:59–68.

22 Pollmann W, Feneberg W: Current management of pain associated with multiple sclerosis. CNS Drugs 2008;22:291–324.

23 Rog D, Nurmikko T, Friede T, Young C: Randomized, controlled trial of cannabis-based medicine in central pain in multiple sclerosis. Neurology 2005;65: 812–819.

24 Svendsen KB, Jensen TS, Bach FW: Does the cannabinoid dronabinol reduce central pain in multiple sclerosis? Randomised double blind placebo controlled crossover trial. BMJ 2004;329:253.

25 Wade DT, Makela P, Robson P, House H, Bateman C: Do cannabis-based medicinal extracts have general or specific effects on symptoms in multiple sclerosis? A double-blind, randomized, placebo-controlled study on 160 patients. Mult Scler 2004;10:434–441.

26 Wade D, Robson P, House H, Makela P, Aram J: A preliminary controlled study to determine whether whole-plant cannabis extracts can improve intractable neurogenic symptoms. Clin Rehabil 2003;17: 21–29.

27 Maurer M, Henn V, Dittrich A, Hofmann A: Δ^9-Tetrahydrocannabinol shows antispastic and analgesic effects in a single-case double-blind trial. Eur Arch Psychiatry Clin Neurosci 1990;240:1–4.

28 Malfitano AM, Proto MC, Bifulco M: Cannabinoids in the management of spasticity associated with multiple sclerosis. Neuropsychiatr Dis Treat 2008;4: 847–853.

29 Petro DJ, Ellenberger C Jr: Treatment of human spasticity with Δ^9-tetrahydrocannabinol. J Clin Pharmacol 1981;21(8–9 suppl):413S–416S.

30 Ungerleider JT, Andyrsiak T, Fairbanks L, Ellison GW, Myers LW: Δ^9-Tetrahydrocannabinol in the treatment of spasticity associated with multiple sclerosis. Adv Alcohol Subst Abuse 1987;7:39–50.

31 Collin C, Davies P, Mutiboko IK, Ratcliffe S, Sativex Spasticity in MS Study Group: Randomized controlled trial of cannabis-based medicine in spasticity caused by multiple sclerosis. Eur J Neurol 2007; 14:290–296.

32 Wade DT, Makela PM, House H, Bateman C, Robson P: Long-term use of a cannabis-based medicine in the treatment of spasticity and other symptoms in multiple sclerosis. Mult Scler 2006;12: 639–645.

33 Zajicek J, Fox P, Sanders H, Wright D, Vickery J, Nunn A, Thompson A, UK MS Research Group: Cannabinoids for treatment of spasticity and other symptoms related to multiple sclerosis (CAMS study): multicenter randomised placebo-controlled trial. Lancet 2003;362:1517–1526.

34 Killestein J, Hoogervorst EL, Reif M, Kalkers NF, van Loenen AC, Staats PG, Gorter RW, Uitdehaag BM, Polman CH: Safety, tolerability, and efficacy of orally administered cannabinoids in MS. Neurology 2002;58:1404–1407.

35 Wissel J, Haydn R, Müller J, Brenneis C, Berger T, Poewe W, Schelosky LD: Low-dose treatment with the synthetic cannabinoid nabilone significantly reduces spasticity-related pain: a double-blind placebo-controlled cross-over trial. J Neurol 2006; 253:1337–1341.

36 Vaney C, Heinzel-Gutenbrunner M, Jobin P, Tschopp F, Gattlen B, Hagen U, Schnelle M, Reif M: Efficacy, safety and tolerability of an orally administered cannabis extract in the treatment of spasticity in patients with multiple sclerosis: a randomized, double-blind, placebo-controlled, crossover study. Mult Scler 2004;10:417–424.

37 Hagenbach U, Luz S, Ghafoor N, Berger JM, Grotenhermen F, Brenneisen R, Mäder M: The treatment of spasticity with Δ^9-tetrahydrocannabinol in persons with spinal cord injury. Spinal Cord 2007;45:551–562.

38 Noyes R Jr, Brunk SF, Avery DA, Canter AC: The analgesic properties of Δ^9-tetrahydrocannabinol and codeine. Clin Pharmacol Ther 1975;15: 139–143.

39 Wilsey B, Marcotte T, Tsodikov A, Millman J, Bentley H, Gouaux B, Fishman S: A randomized, placebo-controlled, crossover trial of cannabis cigarettes in neuropathic pain. J Pain 2008;9: 506–521.

40 Frank B, Serpell MG, Hughes J, Matthews JN, Kapur D: Comparison of analgesic effects and patient tolerability of nabilone and dihydrocodeine for chronic neuropathic pain: randomised, crossover, double blind study. BMJ 2008;336:199–201.

41 Notcutt W, Price M, Miller R, Newport S, Phillips C, Simmons S, Sansom C: Initial experiences with medicinal extracts of cannabis for chronic pain: results from 34 'N of 1' studies. Anaesthesia 2004;59: 440–452.

42 Karst M, Salim K, Burstein S, Conrad I, Hoy L, Schneider U: Analgesic effect of the synthetic cannabinoid CT-3 on chronic neuropathic pain. JAMA 2003;290:1757–1762.

43 Berman JS, Symonds C, Birch R: Efficacy of two cannabis-based medicinal extracts for relief of central neuropathic pain from brachial plexus avulsion: results of a randomized controlled trial. Pain 2004; 112:299–306.

44 Hall W, Solowij N: Adverse effects of cannabis. Lancet 1998;352:1611–1616.

45 Wang T, Collet JP, Shapiro S, Ware MA: Adverse effects of medical cannabinoids: a systematic review. CMAJ 2008;178:1669–1678.

46 Institute of Medicine: Marijuana and medicine: assessing the science base. Washington, National Academy Press, 1999.

47 Degenhardt L, Hall WD: The adverse effects of cannabinoids: implications for use of medical marijuana. CMAJ 2008;178:1685–1686.

48 Cohen SP: Cannabinoids for chronic pain. BMJ 2008;336:167–168.

49 Tetrault JM, Crothers K, Moore BA, Mehra R, Concato J, Fiellin DA: Effects of marijuana smoking on pulmonary function and respiratory complications: a systematic review. Arch Intern Med 2007; 167:221–228.

50 Fernandez-Espejo E, Viveros M, Nuñez L, Ellenbroek BA, Rodriguez de Fonseca F: Role of cannabis and endocannabinoids in the genesis of schizophrenia. Psychopharmacology (Berl) 2009; 206:531–549.

51 le Bec PY, Fatséas M, Denis C, Lavie E, Auriacombe M: Cannabis and psychosis: search of a casual link through a critical and systematic review (in French). Encephale 2009;35:377–385.

52 Lichtman AH, Martin BR: Cannabinoid tolerance and dependence. Handb Exp Pharmacol 2005;168: 691–717.

53 Kalant H: Adverse effects of cannabis on health: an update of the literature since 1996. Prog Neuropsychopharmacol Biol Psychiatry 2004;28: 849–863.

54 Hartman CA, Hopfer CJ, Haberstick B, Rhee SH, Crowley TJ, Corley RP, Hewitt JK, Ehringer MA: The association between cannabinoid receptor 1 gene (CNR1) and cannabis dependence symptoms in adolescents and young adults. Drug Alcohol Depend 2009;104:11–16.

55 Zuo L, Kranzler HR, Luo X: CNR1 variation modulates risk for drug and alcohol dependence. Biol Psychiatry 2007;62:616–626.

56 Zajicek JP, Sanders HP, Wright DE, Vickery PJ, Ingram WM, Reilly SM, Nunn AJ, Teare LJ, Fox PJ, Thompson AJ: Cannabinoids in Multiple Sclerosis (CAMS) study: safety and efficacy data for 12 months follow-up. J Neurol Neurosurg Psychiatry 2005;76:1664–1669.

Steven P. Cohen, MD
Johns Hopkins Pain Management Division
550 North Broadway, Suite 301
Baltimore, MD 21029 (USA)
Tel. +1 410 955 1818, E-Mail scohen40@jhmi.edu

Clark MR, Treisman GJ (eds): Chronic Pain and Addiction.
Adv Psychosom Med. Basel, Karger, 2011, vol 30, pp 139–161

Ketamine in Pain Management

Steven P. Cohen[a,c] · Wesley Liao[a] · Anita Gupta[b] ·
Anthony Plunkett[d]

[a]Pain Management Division, Department of Anesthesiology and Critical Care Medicine,
Johns Hopkins School of Medicine, Baltimore, Md., [b]Pain Management Division, Department of Anesthesiology,
University of Pennsylvania School of Medicine, Philadelphia, Pa., and [c]Department of Surgery and [d]Anesthesia
Service, Department of Surgery, Walter Reed Army Medical Center, Washington, D.C., USA

Abstract

Ketamine is an *N*-methyl-D-aspartate receptor antagonist that has been in clinical use in the USA
for over 30 years. Its ability to provide profound analgesia and amnesia while maintaining spontaneous respiration makes it an ideal medication for procedure-related pain and trauma. In the
chronic pain arena, its use continues to evolve. There is strong evidence to support its short-term
use for neuropathic and nociceptive pain, and conflicting evidence for preemptive analgesia. Its
potential ability to prevent 'windup' and, possibly, 'reboot' aberrant neurologic pathways in neuropathic and central pain states has generated intense interest. However, the long-term use of
ketamine for chronic neuropathic pain is limited by its side effect profile, and is largely anecdotal.
More research is needed to better ascertain its long-term efficacy and side effects, to determine
the ideal candidates for sustained treatment and to develop means of exploiting the antinociceptive properties of ketamine while minimizing the adverse effects.

Copyright © 2011 S. Karger AG, Basel

Ketamine is a medication characterized by a multitude of clinical properties effected
through myriad receptors. Via its antagonistic effects at the *N*-methyl-D-aspartate
(NMDA) receptor, ketamine possesses profound analgesic properties, but also has the
ability to produce hypnosis and amnesia, which likely results from complex interactions at multiple receptor subtypes. First used clinically in the USA in 1970, the role
of ketamine as a common analgesic agent has been limited due to its potential for psychomimetic effects. However, its unique dual properties as an anesthetic agent with
powerful antinociceptive effects, and its ability to prevent or even reverse 'windup',
make it a useful tool in refractory chronic pain states characterized by central sensitization and neuroplasticity.

Brief History

Most commonly classified as an NMDA receptor antagonist, ketamine was first developed by Dr. Craig Newlands of Wayne State University, and subsequently synthesized by Calvin Stevens at Parke-Davis in 1962. Ketamine induces a state of dissociative anesthesia, similar to phencyclidine (PCP), which acts at the same binding site on the NMDA receptor complex. In fact, its developmental inspiration came from the need for a safer anesthetic alternative to PCP, the undesirable side effect profile of which includes hallucinations, neurotoxicity and seizures. Although ketamine was officially released for clinical use in the USA in 1970, it was widely used as a field anesthetic by the US Army during the Vietnam War. It is still used today as a battlefield anesthetic, in mass casualty disasters and for out-of-hospital emergencies. Ketamine continues to be employed in veterinary medicine, particularly for small animals, and during equine surgery (where is it used as the primary intravenous anesthetic agent). In 1999, ketamine became a Schedule III substance under the Controlled Substances Act.

Mechanism of Action

Ketamine likely exerts its effects on the hippocampal formation and prefrontal cortex. Its mechanism of action is primarily by inhibition of NMDA receptors as a noncompetitive antagonist. The NMDA receptor is a ligand-gated channel for which the major endogenous agonist is glutamate, the predominant excitatory neurotransmitter in the central nervous system. Inhibition at this receptor results in decreased neuronal activity. Activation of the NMDA channel is thought to be the major contributor to the 'windup' phenomenon. Hence, antagonism at this receptor may be especially beneficial in chronic pathological pain states characterized by central sensitization and neuroplasticity [1, 2].

Low-dose ketamine administration exerts 'antihyperalgesic and antiallodynic' effects via NMDA receptor antagonism. In higher doses, ketamine (full anesthetic doses) results in activation of different types of opioid receptors with various affinities (μ-, κ-, σ-opioids) [3, 4]. However, the antinociceptive effects of ketamine are not reversed by naloxone, which suggests that its interactions with opioid receptors are not the primary source of analgesia [3, 5]. The protean pharmacological properties of ketamine may also be due its ability to act on a multitude of receptor systems, which includes antagonistic effects on nicotinic and muscarinic acetylcholine receptors, voltage-gated calcium channels [1], local anesthetic effects secondary to its ability to block sodium channels, agonism at high-affinity D_2 dopamine receptors [6], and the facilitation of γ-aminobutyric acid ($GABA_A$) signaling.

Ketamine exists as a racemic mixture comprised of R(−)- and S(+)-stereoisomers. The S(+)-stereoisomer has approximately 3–4 times greater anesthetic potency than its R(−) counterpart due to its higher affinity for the PCP binding site of the NMDA receptor [1]. Compared to racemic ketamine, the S(+)-stereoisomer is significantly shorter acting, induces more drowsiness, and possesses greater analgesic properties despite less hallucinogenic side effects. The R(–)-stereoisomer is a stronger σ-agonist than racemic ketamine, which likely contributes to the decreased seizure threshold observed with ketamine.

Ketamine is unique in that no other drug in clinical practice exhibits the combination of hypnotic, analgesic and amnestic effects. The hypnotic effects may be due to inhibition of hyperpolarization-activated cyclic nucleotide-modulated (HCN1) nonspecific cation channels that mediate 'sag' currents which help stabilize membrane potential and regulate spike frequency [7]. The mechanisms of the amnestic effects of ketamine are still not well elucidated, but are likely to result from interactions at a multitude of receptors including NMDA, serotonin and nicotinic acetylcholine [8, 9].

Pharmacokinetics and Pharmacodynamics

Ketamine is most commonly available as a white crystalline powder, liquid or tablet. It may be administered via many routes including intravenously, intramuscularly, by insufflation/intranasally, by inhalation (smoked), orally (elixir), topically (little to no systemic absorption) and rectally. Ketamine is water and lipid soluble, which allows for extensive distribution in the body and rapid crossing of the blood-brain barrier. It is rapidly distributed in the brain and other highly perfused tissues, while approximately 12% remains protein bound in plasma [10]. The metabolism of ketamine is mediated by hepatic microsomal enzymes, most notably cytochrome P450. Orally ingested ketamine is rapidly metabolized to norketamine and dehydronorketamine [10]. The excretion of ketamine and its metabolites is via urine.

In low doses, ketamine causes analgesia and sedation, while in high doses, it produces general anesthesia. The clinical effects of ketamine include an increase in cerebral blood flow and metabolism in spontaneously breathing patients [10]. The stimulating effects of ketamine on the cardiovascular system mostly stem from stimulation of the sympathetic nervous system. The direct myocardial depressant effects are typically only realized in catecholamine-depleted individuals (e.g. long-term trauma or intensive care patients). The resultant increase in blood pressure and heart rate, coupled with its ability to cause bronchodilation, make it an ideal drug for trauma victims in the setting of hypovolemia, septic shock or pulmonary disease. The dissociative anesthetic properties of ketamine are thought to result from a combination of reduced activation of the thalamocortical system and increased activity in the limbic system and hippocampus [10]. Analgesia from ketamine usually ensues when plasma concentrations approach 100 ng/ml [10]. One advantage over opioid therapy is that long-term ketamine use is associated with minimal, if any, tolerance and tachyphylaxis [11, 12] (table 1).

Table 1. Pharmacokinetics of ketamine administration for different routes

Route of administration	Typical dosing	Bioavailability	Onset	Duration of action
Intravenous	1–2 mg/kg for general anesthesia induction; 1–6 mg/kg/h for anesthesia maintenance; 0.4–0.75 mg/kg/h for 3–5 days awake ketamine infusions for chronic neuropathic pain; 0.2–1.0 mg/kg for procedural analgesia; 0.1/mg/kg for i.v. infusion test; 1–4 mg/demand dose mixed with opioids in PCA for postoperative pain, or 5–15 mg/h when infused separately	N/A	<30 s	30–45 min after bolus dosing
Intramuscular	2–4 × i.v. dosing; 5–10 mg/kg for surgical anesthesia	90%	1–5 min	30–75 min
Intranasal	0.2–0.5 mg/kg for chronic pain and sedation; 3–6 mg/kg for procedural analgesia and anesthetic premedication	25–50%	5–10 min	45–60 min
Subcutaneous	0.05–0.15 mg/kg/h for chronic neuropathic pain	> 75%	5–10 min	N/A
Oral	0.3–1 mg/kg for chronic pain; up to 3 mg/kg for procedural analgesia and anesthetic premedication	10–20%	15–20 min	1–2 h
Rectal	5–10 mg/kg for anesthesia premedication and procedural analgesia	25–30%	5–15 min	2–3 h
Topical	0.5–10% cream	<5%	<2 days	N/A

PCA = Patient-controlled analgesia.

Evidence for Analgesic Efficacy

Opioids are the cornerstone of acute perioperative pain management. However, neurophysiological mechanisms of analgesia extend beyond opioid receptor agonism. A growing body of scientific literature describes nonopioid-related alterations in inhibitory and excitatory pathways mediated by windup phenomena, neurokinins and the NMDA receptor [10]. Among nonopioid agents, ketamine has demonstrated evidence for analgesic efficacy in both supplemental as well as stand-alone treatment. In clinical settings, ketamine is often given as a low-dose bolus or parenteral infusion, as a supplement to opioid-based analgesia to treat inflammatory pain. It has also been used as a 'rescue agent' in patients with opioid-refractory, acute postoperative pain.

Ketamine and Opioids

In rodent models, subanesthetic doses of ketamine have been shown to prevent the development of hyperalgesia and tolerance observed with opioid administration [13]. In human experimental models, low-dose ketamine was demonstrated to prevent the long-term increase in perceived pain due to electrical test stimuli induced by high-frequency electrical stimulation of nociceptive afferents in humans [14]. In a small study conducted on human volunteers exposed to a skin burn injury on the leg, synergistic analgesic effects were found with coadministration of ketamine and morphine on pain involving central sensitization phenomena [15]. A prospective randomized study assessing the use of low-dose ketamine as an adjunct in opioid-tolerant patients for 24 h after spinal fusion found decreased postoperative pain and a trend towards decreased opioid requirements in the treatment group when compared to control patients [16]. One possible mechanism for ketamine synergism with opioids is that NMDA stimulation and downstream messengers have been implicated in the development of opioid tolerance and physical dependence [17].

Ketamine has been used as an adjunct to opioid therapy in patients treated with patient-controlled analgesia (PCA) for postoperative pain. Numerous studies have demonstrated that the addition of ketamine to intravenous morphine PCA results in decreased opioid requirements in the first 24 h after surgery. One study found opioid consumption was reduced by about 30%, with diminished nausea and vomiting [18]. However, systematic reviews have been mixed. In a Cochrane Database review, the addition of ketamine to intravenous opioid PCA led to reductions in postoperative pain intensity or opioid requirements in 27 out of 37 trials, with only mild or absent adverse effects [18]. But in an earlier review, Subramaniam et al. [19] concluded that the addition of low-dose ketamine to morphine PCA does not improve analgesia. Ketamine PCA has also been used as a stand-alone treatment in chronic pain patients with extreme opioid tolerance [2]. Other potential benefits of adding ketamine to opioid PCA may be more rapid improvement in functional capacity [20], and reduced respiratory dysfunction [21]. When ketamine is combined with morphine PCA, most studies have used ratios on the order of 1:1.

Ketamine also enhances the effects of opioid analgesia when administered separately from PCA. A systematic review by Subramaniam et al. [19] found that perioperative intravenous ketamine either reduced pain or opioid requirements when administered as a continuous infusion or in bolus doses. However, when administered in conjunction with epidural opioids, only 2 of 4 trials demonstrated a benefit. In patients with burn injuries, the cardiorespiratory stimulant effects of ketamine, coupled with its ability to provide excellent analgesia for dressing changes and debridements when administered in bolus dosing, and to relieve basal pain when given in low-dose infusions, has made the drug a first-line treatment [22].

Several studies have examined the effects of ketamine use in specific surgeries. Most [23–25] but not all [26] studies have yielded positive findings. In patients undergoing laparotomy, intraoperative ketamine continued for 48 h postoperatively was found to reduce opioid-induced hyperalgesia associated with remifentanil infusion [23]. Double-blind studies have also found that perioperative ketamine reduces wound hyperalgesia after nephrectomy [24] and laparotomy [25]. In a review by de Kock and Lavand'homme [27], the authors concluded that ketamine is an effective means of reducing postoperative hyperalgesia associated with opioid-administered and trauma-induced central sensitization.

Nociceptive Pain
The use of ketamine in conditions involving nociceptive pain has also been investigated. One placebo-controlled study found no significant benefit resulted from intra-articular injection of ketamine in patients with temporomandibular disorder, suggesting that peripheral NMDA receptors do not play a significant role in this condition [28]. For fibromyalgia, the results have been more positive. Randomized controlled studies have suggested that central NMDA receptors may play a primary role in fibromyalgia, as evidenced by a significant reduction in symptoms among a large proportion of patients in response to ketamine [29, 30]. However, the 0.3 mg/kg dose administered in these studies may have undermined the NMDA selectivity of the infusion, such that pain relief could have resulted from the dissociative effects. Since no etiologic tissue pathology has been reliably identified in fibromyalgia, many experts feel the condition is best classified as a form of central, rather than nociceptive, pain. In a recent review, Wood [31] suggested that the beneficial effect of ketamine in fibromyalgia may stem from stimulation of high-affinity dopamine receptors in the limbic system.

Alternative Delivery Systems
Oral and intranasal ketamine have been investigated in the treatment of chronic pain. In a double-blind, placebo-controlled crossover study, Carr et al. [32] found that intranasal ketamine administered in 10-mg increments resulted in modest-breakthrough pain reduction compared to placebo for up to 1 h after the initial dose in 20 patients with mostly nociceptive pain. In a subsequent randomized study performed on patients with neuropathic pain, both 0.2 mg/kg and 0.4 mg/kg significantly reduced pain scores, with no dose-response relationship noted [33]. The results for oral ketamine are even less auspicious, with two randomized controlled studies demonstrating mixed results [34, 35]. The major downside of long-term intranasal and chronic ketamine is the high incidence of side effects.

Ketamine has occasionally been used as an adjuvant to other analgesic agents given neuraxially. There are numerous anecdotal reports touting the beneficial effects of administering intrathecal ketamine to terminal cancer patients unresponsive to conventional intrathecal therapy [36, 37]. In a double-blind crossover study, Yang et al. [38] compared the coadministration of low-dose intrathecal ketamine (1 mg) plus morphine with morphine alone twice daily in 20 patients with terminal cancer. The authors found that combination treatment resulted in significantly lower opioid requirements, less rescue medication and slightly improved pain scores compared with morphine alone over the 48-hour treatment period, with no serious side effects. In a randomized, double-blind, placebo-controlled study comparing epidural ketamine-bupivacaine with bupivacaine alone, started preoperatively and continued for 48–72 h postoperatively for lower limb amputation, Wilson et al. [39] found that the ketamine group experienced superior postoperative analgesia compared with the control group. However, no differences were noted with respect to the incidence rates of stump or phantom pain between groups over the 1-year follow-up period. In light of concerns regarding neurotoxicity with neuraxial administration [40], the use of spinal ketamine should be reserved for terminal patients who have failed to derive relief from safer and more conventional analgesic regimens [41].

Ketamine has been used in topical form as an adjuvant for neuropathic pain. In a recent double-blind, placebo-controlled crossover trial conducted on 20 patients with complex regional pain syndrome (CRPS), racemic ketamine hydrochloride 10% cream reduced brush allodynia and, to a lesser extent, punctuate hyperalgesia 30 min after application in the affected extremity compared with placebo [42]. However, no reduction in spontaneous pain was observed. Because neither ketamine nor its metabolite, norketamine, were detected in plasma samples, and topical application to the unaffected extremity did not result in symptom palliation in the affected limb, the authors concluded that the mechanism of action involved antagonism of peripheral NMDA receptors. In another randomized study comparing the topical administration of ketamine and morphine in children after tonsillectomy, Canbay et al. [43] found that ketamine and morphine as stand-alone treatments and in combination were more effective in the first hour after administration than placebo. Interestingly, the duration of action of each treatment given individually was longer than in combination. Whereas randomized trials evaluating topical ketamine show promise in patients with evoked pain (i.e. allodynia and hyperalgesia), there is limited evidence supporting its use for spontaneous pain and in patients with multifocal symptomatology.

In children, ketamine is used in high relative doses (compared with adults) to provide effective sedation for painful procedures, with fewer side effects than opioid-based techniques [44]. Oral, intranasal and rectal ketamine are frequently used as premedicants in anxious children, and intramuscular administration is commonly employed for anesthesia in uncooperative pediatric patients without intravenous access. In view of its physiological effects, it is frequently chosen for anesthetic induction in patients with cyanotic conditions and neuromuscular disorders, who are at increased risk for malignant hypothermia [45, 46].

Neuropathic Pain
Ketamine is considered a potential treatment option in neuropathic pain patients who have failed conventional therapy. Most frequently, it is employed to treat CRPS, a regional pain disorder characterized by sensory, autonomic, motor and dystrophic signs/symptoms outside of the distribution of a single nerve. It is hypothesized that

ketamine works via manipulation of NMDA receptors that may reboot aberrant activity in the central nervous system, resulting in 'unwinding' of central sensitization and, ultimately, a reduction in spontaneous and evoked pain.

For the treatment of CRPS, several treatment modalities have been described. The first is a low-dose outpatient infusion. In a double-blind, placebo-controlled study, Schwartzman et al. [47] randomized 19 patients to receive either ketamine 0.35 mg/kg/h or saline for 4 h per day over 10 days. During the 12-week follow-up, patients in the ketamine group exhibited modest decreases in spontaneous pain, but no improvement in quality of life. Whether true 'blinding' can be accomplished with ketamine infusions is a question that remains to be answered. In a similar study by Goldberg et al. [48], the authors reported that infusions of escalating doses of ketamine from 40 to 80 mg over a 10-day period were associated with significant improvements in pain and the ability to initiate movement. No outcomes were assessed after cessation of the infusion. The second method of infusion is an awake continuous infusion as an inpatient. In a retrospective study by Correll et al. [49], 33 patients underwent inpatient ketamine infusion (mean dose: 23.4 mg/h) over an average period of 4.7 days. After the initial treatment, 76% of the patients obtained complete, and 25% experienced partial pain relief, with the benefit lasting more than 3 months in over half the subjects. Among the 12 patients who received a second infusion, 58% obtained excellent relief lasting more than 1 year. A variation on this technique involves the induction of a high-dose (3–5 mg/kg/h) ketamine coma over an approximately 5-day period. Although complete remission has been reported with this therapy, it requires mechanical ventilation and is associated with significant risks. In addition to CRPS, other forms of neuropathic pain that have been treated with ketamine infusions include lumbar radiculopathy and postherpetic neuralgia.

Central Pain

There is also strong evidence to support the short-term use of ketamine for central pain, which tends to be more resistant to treatment than peripheral neuropathic pain. A randomized controlled crossover study by Eide et al. [50] found that low-dose ketamine (6 μg/kg/min after a bolus dose of 60 μg/kg) and alfentanil significantly reduced continuous and evoked pain in 9 patients with central dysesthetic pain following spinal cord injury. In a later study utilizing somewhat higher subanesthetic doses (0.4 mg/kg bolus), Kvarnström et al. [51] reported that ketamine, but not lidocaine or placebo, reduced neuropathic pain beneath the level of injury in 10 spinal cord-injured patients. Double-blind, placebo-controlled studies have also demonstrated short-term efficacy for ketamine in phantom limb pain (n = 20; 0.4 mg/kg) [52] and central pain [50] (tables 2, 3).

Preemptive Analgesia

The goals of preemptive analgesia include decreasing the intensity and duration of acute pain after tissue injury, preventing pain-related pathological modulation of the central nervous system, and reducing the incidence of chronic pain [79]. But whereas animal models clearly support the concept of preemptive analgesia, the clinical

Table 2. Randomized controlled studies evaluating ketamine for chronic pain

Study	Study design	Patients	Medications	Results
Schwartzman et al. [47]	Randomized, double-blind, placebo-controlled	26 patients with CRPS	10 days; 4 h i.v. ketamine infusion vs. placebo; max. infusion rate: 0.35 mg/kg/h; average ketamine plasma level: 188.4 ng/ml	Ketamine >placebo; significance lost at 3-month follow-up
Finch et al. [42]	Double-blind, placebo-controlled	20 consecutive patients with CRPS	Topical application of 0.5 ml of 10% ketamine or placebo	Ketamine > placebo through 1-week follow-up
Sigtermans et al. [53]	Double-blind, randomized, placebo-controlled, parallel-group	60 patients with CRPS type I	Ketamine infusion of 4.2 days; average dose: 22.2 mg/h/70 kg	Ketamine > placebo over 12-week follow-up
Castrillon et al. [54]	Double-blind, randomized, placebo-controlled	14 patients with myogenous temporomandibular disorder	0.2 ml of 10 mmol/l ketamine or saline injected into the masseter muscle	Ketamine = saline up to 24 h after injection
Eichenberger et al. [52]	Randomized, double-blind, crossover	20 patients with chronic phantom limb pain	Infusions of calcitonin 200 IU, 0.4 mg/kg ketamine (10 patients), calcitonin plus ketamine, or saline	Ketamine-calcitonin and ketamine alone > calcitonin and placebo up to 1 h after infusion; combination > placebo up to 48 h after infusion
Lemming et al. [55]	Double-blind, randomized, placebo-controlled crossover	20 patients with chronic whiplash-associated pain	Infusions of placebo-placebo, ketamine-placebo, remifentanil-placebo or ketamine-remifentanil in crossover fashion; ketamine plasma concentration: 100 ng/ml	Ketamine-remifentanil > ketamine-placebo and remifentanil-placebo > placebo up to 65 min after infusion

Table 2. Continued

Study	Study design	Patients	Medications	Results
Gottrup et al. [56]	2 randomized, double-blind, placebo-controlled, crossover studies	20 patients with neuropathic pain	On 4 different days, patients received a 30-min i.v. infusion of ketamine (0.24 mg/kg), lidocaine (5 mg/kg) or saline	Ketamine > lidocaine > placebo; no long-term follow-up
Lynch et al. [57]	Double-blind, randomized, placebo-controlled	92 patients with diabetic neuropathy, postherpetic neuralgia or postsurgical/ posttraumatic neuropathic pain	Topical placebo, 2% amitriptyline, 1% ketamine or amitriptyline-ketamine combination q.i.d.	No difference between groups through 3-week follow-up
Carr et al. [32]	Randomized, double-blind, placebo-controlled, crossover	20 patients with breakthrough pain due to various chronic pain conditions	Intranasal 10% ketamine (up to 50 mg) or placebo	Ketamine > placebo; no long-term follow-up
Kvarnström et al. [51]	Randomized, double-blind, 3-period, crossover	10 patients with central pain after spinal cord injury	I.v. ketamine 0.4 mg/kg, lidocaine 2.5 mg/kg or placebo, infused over 40 min	Ketamine > lidocaine and placebo; no long-term follow-up
Jørum et al. [58]	Randomized, double-blind, placebo-controlled, crossover	12 patients with neuropathic pain	I.v. ketamine 60 µg/ kg bolus, then infusion of 6 mg/ kg/min, i.v. alfentanil 7 µg/kg bolus, then infusion of 0.6 mg/kg/min, or placebo over 20 min	Alfentanil = ketamine > placebo; no long-term follow-up
Lynch et al. [59]	2-day, randomized, double-blind, placebo-controlled, 4-way crossover	20 patients with chronic neuropathic pain	Topical 1% amitriptyline, 0.5% ketamine, ketamine-amitriptyline combination or placebo	No difference from placebo after 2 days for any treatment

Table 2. Continued

Study	Study design	Patients	Medications	Results
Leung et al. [60]	Randomized, double-blind	12 patients with neuropathic pain after nerve injury	I.v. infusion titrated to alfentanil at 25, 50 and 75 ng/ml, ketamine at 50, 100 and 150 ng/ml, or a diphenhydramine placebo	Alfentanil = ketamine > placebo for cold pain thresholds; no long-term follow-up
Graven-Nielsen et al. [30]	Double-blind, placebo-controlled, crossover	29 female patients with fibromyalgia	I.v. ketamine 0.3 mg/kg or placebo over 30 min	Ketamine > placebo through 150-min follow-up
Mercadante et al. [61]	Randomized, controlled, double-blind, crossover	10 patients with chronic cancer pain	I.v. ketamine 0.25 mg/kg or 0.50 mg/kg, or placebo on 3 separate days	High-dose ketamine > low-dose ketamine > placebo over 3 h after infusion
Lauretti et al. [62]	Randomized, double-blind	48 terminal cancer pain patients	Control group received 2 mg epidural morphine twice daily vs. combination of morphine plus 0.2 mg/kg ketamine, morphine plus 100 μg neostigmine, or morphine plus 500 μg midazolam	Ketamine-morphine combination > other groups through 25-day follow-up
Rabben et al. [63]	Randomized, double-blind, comparative-effectiveness crossover followed by randomized, double-blind, placebo-controlled	30 patients with trigeminal neuropathic pain	I.m. injection of ketamine 0.4 mg/kg plus midazolam or pethidine 1.0 mg/kg; 1 week later, patients received either 4.0 mg/kg ketamine or placebo q.h.s. over 3 days	Ketamine > pethidine after i.m. injection; ketamine > placebo for up to 3 days after oral administration; no long-term follow-up
Persson et al. [64]	Randomized, double-blind, cross-over	8 patients with rest pain due to arteriosclerosis obliterans	Ketamine at 0.15, 0.30 or 0.45 mg/kg and morphine 10 mg as a 5-min infusion on 4 separate days	Ketamine at highest dose (0.45 mg/kg) > morphine; no long-term follow-up

Table 2. Continued

Study	Study design	Patients	Medications	Results
Nikolajsen et al. [65]	Randomized, double-blind, crossover	11 patients with postamputation stump and phantom limb pain	Ketamine bolus of 0.1 mg/kg, followed by i.v. infusion at 7 μg/kg/min for 45 min or placebo	Ketamine > placebo for postamputation stump and phantom limb pain over 80 min; no long-term follow-up
Felsby et al. [66]	Double-blind, placebo-controlled	10 patients with peripheral neuropathic pain	I.v. ketamine 0.2 mg/kg, i.v. magnesium 0.16 mmol/kg bolus, then an infusion of ketamine 0.3 mg/kg/h, vs. magnesium 0.16 mmol/kg/h for a total of 1 h; plasma ketamine levels not measured	Ketamine > magnesium for spontaneous pain; no long-term follow-up
Max et al. [67]	Randomized, placebo-controlled, double-blind, crossover	8 patients with chronic posttraumatic pain and allodynia	2-hour i.v. infusions of ketamine (mean dose: 58 mg), alfentanil (mean dose: 11 mg) or placebo	Ketamine > alfentanil and placebo; no long-term follow-up
Nicolodi and Sicuteri [68]	Randomized, double-blind, cross-over	17 patients with migraine	Ketamine 80 μg/kg s.c. 3 times a day or saline randomly assigned in a 3-week chronic treatment	Ketamine > placebo; no long-term follow-up
Eide et al. [50]	Randomized, double-blind, crossover	9 patients with central dysesthesia pain after traumatic spinal cord injury	Infusions of ketamine 6 μg/kg/min, alfentanil 0.6 μg/kg/min and placebo in crossover fashion for 17–21 min; median ketamine plasma concentration: 110 ng/ml	Ketamine > alfentanil and placebo; no long-term follow-up

Table 2. Continued

Study	Study design	Patients	Medications	Results
Eide et al. [69]	Randomized, double-blind, crossover	8 patients with postherpetic neuralgia	I.v. infusion of ketamine 0.15 mg/kg, morphine 0.075 mg/kg, or placebo over 10 min	Ketamine = morphine > placebo; ketamine = morphine for pain scores; ketamine > morphine for allodynia and windup; no long-term follow-up
Backonja et al. [70]	Double-blind, placebo-controlled	3 patients with peripheral neuropathic pain, and 3 with central pain	2 ketamine boluses of 250 µg/kg or placebo; 2 patients were given additional boluses	5/6 patients had pain relief with ketamine but not placebo over 2–3 h; no long-term follow-up

evidence garnered from systematic reviews is conflicting, either showing no preemptive analgesia or only marginal benefit [79–81]. A recent meta-analysis by Ong et al. [82] demonstrated poor efficacy for the preemptive effects of intravenous ketamine before surgery on both postoperative pain scores and analgesic usage. Subsequent attempts to evaluate the ability of ketamine to diminish postsurgical pain have for the most part been similarly disappointing [83–88].

In view of the high incidence of adverse effects with long-term ketamine administration, attempts have been made to use it diagnostically to identify pain mechanisms, and prognostically to predict the longer-term response to other NMDA receptor antagonists. The rationale for low-dose infusion tests to identify cellular mechanisms of nociception is based on the premise that mechanistic treatment of pain may be superior to etiology-based therapy [89]. Scandinavian investigators have employed double-blind crossover studies using 0.3 mg/kg ketamine to determine that NMDA receptors may play a role in fibromyalgia [90, 91]. Follow-up studies utilizing SPECT scans after ketamine administration to fibromyalgia patients have shown that changes in regional brain perfusion patterns may predict response to ketamine [92].

Cohen et al. [93–95] recently conducted a series of correlational studies to determine whether an ultralow dose of ketamine (0.1 mg/kg), which would presumably act selectively at NMDA receptors, could predict the subsequent response to a 6- to 8-week treatment regimen with the oral NMDA receptor antagonist dextromethorphan in patients with neuropathic pain, fibromyalgia and opioid tolerance. When data from all 3 studies were combined, the collective sensitivity, specificity, positive predictive value

Table 3. Clinical studies evaluating long-term use of ketamine for chronic pain

Study	Study design	Patients	Medications	Results
Huge et al. [33]	Randomized, open-label	16 patients with neuropathic pain	2 treatment groups: intranasal S-ketamine 0.2 mg/kg vs. S-ketamine 0.4 mg/kg (group 2)	Pain scores decreased significantly in both groups, with min. pain at 60 min after drug administration; no long-term follow-up
Ryan et al. [71]	Retrospective chart review	8 patients with refractory mucositis pain	Ketamine swish and swallow (20 mg/5 ml) every 4 h as needed; average duration: 6 days	Pain reduced in 5/8 patients; no pain scores recorded or long-term follow-up
Kiefer et al. [72]	Open-label	20 patients with CRPS	Patients were intubated with a bolus of ketamine (1–1.5 mg/kg) and midazolam; ketamine infusion given over 5 days titrating up to 7 mg/kg/h	Pain scores decreased from 8.9 to 0.5 at 1 month, and to 2.0 at 6 months
Finkel et al. [73]	Case series	11 children and adolescents with chronic cancer pain	I.v. infusion ranging from 0.1 to 1 mg/kg/h up to 75 days	Significant pain improvement, and reduction in opioid requirement; no long-term follow-up
Webster and Walker [74]	Retrospective chart review	13 patients with nonmalignant neuropathic pain	I.v. or subcutaneous ketamine infusions (mean dose: 0.12 mg/kg/h) for up to 8 weeks (mean: 16.4 days)	Mean pain score decreased from 7.7 at start to 4.8 at end of treatment; no long-term follow-up
Goldberg et al. [48]	Prospective case series	36 male, 4 female patients with CRPS	10-day outpatient i.v. ketamine infusions titrated from 40 mg/day to 80 mg/day	Mean pain score decreased from 7.5 to 5.4 on day 10; no long-term follow-up

Table 3. Continued

Study	Study design	Patients	Medications	Results
Correll et al. [49]	Retrospective chart review	33 patients with CRPS	I.v. ketamine infusion ranging from 15 to 50 mg/h; duration ranged from 0.75 to 20 days	Complete pain relief in 76%, and partial relief in 18% of patients after initial course; 12 patients underwent 2nd or 3rd course; 54% were pain free for >3 months, 31% for >6 months; after 2nd infusion, 58% of patients experienced relief for >1 year
Furuhashi-Yonaha et al. [34]	Randomized, placebo-controlled	8 patients with chronic neuropathic pain who responded to an i.v. ketamine infusion	0.5 mg/kg oral ketamine or placebo q.i.d.	Ketamine > placebo; 4 patients continued to experience long-term (>9-month) benefit
Kannan et al. [75]	Case series	9 patients with neuropathic cancer pain	0.5 mg/kg oral ketamine t.i.d. over 3 days, then every 10 days for 60 days	7/9 patients had pain relief through 60-day follow-up
Kiefer et al. [76]	Case series	6 patients with CRPS	7-day i.v. ketamine infusion titrated up to 7 mg/kg/h	5/6 patients had complete absence of allodynia, hyperalgesia and swelling in affected areas; follow-up ranged from 3 weeks to 2 years
Jackson et al. [77]	Prospective, multicenter, unblinded, open-label audit	39 patients with refractory cancer pain	I.v. ketamine infusion starting at 100 mg/24 h titrated up to max. of 500 mg/24 h	67% of patients showed good pain relief; longest duration of good pain relief was 8 weeks
Lauretti et al. [78]	Prospective, randomized, pilot	60 patients with chronic cancer pain	Oral morphine (10 mg every 12 h) vs. oral ketamine (0.5 mg/kg every 12 h) vs. 5 mg nitroglycerin patch vs. oral Dipyrone 500 mg every 6 h	Only ketamine group > control group at 30-day follow-up for decreased total morphine consumption

Table 3. Continued

Study	Study design	Patients	Medications	Results
Yang et al. [38]	Double-blind, crossover	20 patients with terminal cancer pain	Intrathecal morphine (start at 0.05 mg and titrated up for VAS <4/10) vs. morphine plus ketamine (1.0 mg) twice daily	Ketamine plus morphine > morphine alone for decreased intrathecal opioid requirement; no long-term follow-up

VAS = Visual analog scale.

and negative predictive value were 76, 78, 67 and 85%, respectively. In a systematic review, the evidence supporting the use of intravenous ketamine to predict the response to oral dextromethorphan therapy was considered to be weakly positive [96].

Adverse Effects

Ketamine has a wide therapeutic index. Lethal overdosage with ketamine is unusual, with patients experiencing uneventful recoveries after having inadvertently received 10 times the normal dose [1]. Common adverse effects include hypersalivation, hyper-reflexia, increased muscle tone, transient clonus, emesis and agitation. Stimulation of the sympathetic system typically causes hypertension, tachycardia, and increased intracranial, pulmonary and intraocular pressures, which can have catastrophic consequences in trauma patients [1]. The incidence of laryngospasm requiring airway placement is approximately 1 in 5,000 patients (0.02%) [97].

The most prominent and feared side effects of ketamine are hallucinations and a 'dissociative state'. In recreational users, ketamine can produce severe impairment of working, episodic and semantic memory, and schizotypal and dissociative symptoms. Compared with other hallucinogenic medications, the duration of action is relatively short, lasting less than 90 min depending on the dose and route of administration. These psychotropic effects include sensations such as floating, near-death experiences, and distorted perceptions of time, space and morphology. Multiple studies have demonstrated that the psychotropic effects of ketamine can be reduced by coadministration of benzodiazepines.

The long-term side effects of ketamine on cognition and memory are not well understood. The administration of ketamine clearly diminishes the attention span while the drug is active, but findings are conflicting regarding the long-term effects [98]. Studies conducted on both patients and recreational users demonstrate that ketamine acutely impairs episodic memory acquisition, but leaves memory retrieval (i.e. information obtained before having obtained the drug) largely intact. With regard to semantic memory (general knowledge), the results of studies evaluating acute drug administration are mixed [98]. In chronic ketamine users, research suggests that both episodic and semantic memory deficits can occur [98]. Whereas some cognitive deficits are reversible following cessation of chronic ketamine use [99], others may still be evident years later compared with polydrug control patients [98]. Some experts speculate that the persistent cognitive impairment may be a byproduct of the irreversible cell death observed following repeated high doses of ketamine and other NMDA receptor antagonists [100]. Animal studies show that chronic ketamine use leads to decreased socialization [101, 102].

Many preclinical studies have investigated the effects of ketamine at the cellular level. In 1989, Olney et al. [103] found that ketamine and other noncompetitive NMDA antagonists caused reversible changes in the rat brain. Following subcutaneous administration of 40 mg/kg, which is considerably more than therapeutic dosing in humans, intracellular fluid-filled vacuoles appeared after 4 h, but disappeared after cytopathological examination at day 4. However, no toxicity was noted at lower doses. In later work, the same group found that coadministration of certain anticholinergic or GABAergic agents is protective against the adverse neurotoxic effects of NMDA receptor antagonists.

However, later studies demonstrated conflicting results regarding neurodegenerative effects. Several early investigations found that exposure to ketamine leads to neural apoptosis in the developing rodent brain [104–106]. Subsequent studies performed on primates revealed that long-term (>9-hour) but not short-term exposure to ketamine induced significant brain cell death, and that these effects were most pronounced in newborn animals [107, 108]. Vutskits et al. [109] demonstrated that short-term exposure to ketamine (>20 µg/ml) leads to significant loss of differentiated cells in cell cultures, and that lower doses (10 µg/ml) can precipitate long-term changes in the dendritic arbors of differentiated neurons.

Yet, other studies suggest ketamine and other NMDA receptor antagonists may possess neuroprotective properties. In animal models of ischemia and traumatic brain injury, large doses of ketamine given after injury ameliorate neuronal death [110–113]. A preemptive neuroprotective effect has also been demonstrated in neonatal rat models of inflammatory pain. Anand et al. [114] found that anesthetic doses (5 mg/kg) of ketamine administered before daily formalin injections decreased cell death in newborn rat brains. These seemingly contradictory results suggest that the neurological effects of ketamine may be dependent on species, timing, dose and context, and argue strongly for more research.

Abuse Potential

The first reports of ketamine being used for 'recreational' purposes were on the West Coast of the USA in the 1970s [115]. Over the next 10–15 years, its use as a street drug remained at relatively low levels compared to marijuana, cocaine, opioids and other hallucinogens. Yet, over the past decade its popularity has surged, especially in club goers. A 2007 British survey found that 0.8% of adults aged 18–24 years used ketamine in the past year [116]. Among club drug users, 32% reported using the drug in a 1997 survey; by 2004, this number had ballooned to 43% [117]. In East Asia, ketamine is frequently implicated as a cause of motor vehicle accidents [118–120]. In two studies from Hong Kong, ketamine was found in the systems of 45% of injured drivers involved in nonfatal motor vehicle accidents [119], and in 3% of fatalities [120]. In low doses, ketamine produces distortions of space and time, hallucinations and mild dissociative effects. In higher doses exceeding 1.5 mg/kg, ketamine induces a state commonly referred to as a 'K hole', in which the user experiences an intense detachment from reality [117]. Popular street names for ketamine include 'Special K', 'Vitamin K', 'Kitty Smack' and 'K'.

Conclusions

Ketamine is a potent analgesic that has been used in clinical practice in the USA since the 1970s. Although its primary mechanism of action is via antagonism of the NMDA glutamate receptor, it also acts at a multitude of other binding sites. Ketamine has long served an important role in the perioperative setting, both as an anesthetic agent and for procedural analgesia and sedation. Its role in the management of chronic pain syndromes is relatively new, and stems from its unique potential ability to prevent, or possibly reverse, 'windup'. Whereas compelling evidence exists for short-term benefit in central, peripheral neuropathic and inflammatory pain states, its long-term ability to alleviate pain and improve function is limited by the lack of controlled trials with adequate follow-up, and by the high incidence of psychomimetic effects. More research is needed to establish its long-term efficacy, to find ways to minimize adverse effects, and to determine the ideal conditions and patients for treatment with ketamine, either as a stand-alone analgesic agent or as part of a multidrug treatment regimen.

References

1 Sinner B, Graf BM: Ketamine. Handb Exp Pharmacol 2008;182:313–333.

2 Cohen SP, DeJesus M: Ketamine patient-controlled analgesia for dysesthetic central pain. Spinal Cord 2004;42:425–428.

3 Smith DJ, Bouchal RL, de Sanctis CA, Monroe PJ, Amedro JB, Perrotti JM, Crisp T: Properties of the interaction between ketamine and opiate binding sites in vivo and in vitro. Neuropharmacology 1987; 26:1253–1260.

4 Sarton E, Teppema LLJ, Olievier C, Nieuwenhuijs D, Matthes HW, Kieffer BL, Dahan A: The involvement of the μ-opioid receptor in ketamine-induced respiratory depression and antinociception. Anesth Analg 2001;93:1495–1500.

5 Smith DJ, Perrotti JM, Mansell AL, Monroe PJ: Ketamine analgesia is not related to an opiate action in the periaqueductal gray region of the rat brain. Pain 1985;21:253–265.

6 Seeman P, Ko F, Tallerico T: Dopamine receptor contribution to the action of PCP, LSD and ketamine psychotomimetics. Mol Psychiatry 2005;10: 877–883.

7 Chen X, Shu S, Bayliss D: HCN1 channel subunits are a molecular substrate for hypnotic actions of ketamine. J Neurosci 2009;29:600–609.

8 Coates KM, Flood P: Ketamine and its preservative, benzethonium chloride, both inhibit human recombinant α_7 and $\alpha_4\beta_2$ neuronal nicotinic acetylcholine receptors in *Xenopus* oocytes. Br J Pharmacol 2001; 134:871–879.

9 Liy-Salmeron G, Meneses A: Effects of 5-HT drugs in prefrontal cortex during memory formation and the ketamine amnesia-model. Hippocampus 2008; 18:965–974.

10 Sinner B, Graf BM: Ketamine. Handb Exp Pharmacol 2008;182:313–333.

11 White MC, Karsli C: Long-term use of an intravenous ketamine infusion in a child with significant burns. Paediatr Anaesth 2007;17:1102–1104.

12 Domino EF: Taming the ketamine tiger. 1965. Anesthesiology 2010;113:678–684.

13 Laulin JP, Maurette P, Corcuff JB, Rivat C, Chauvin M, Simonnet G: The role of ketamine in preventing fentanyl-induced hyperalgesia and subsequent acute morphine tolerance. Anesth Analg 2002;94: 1263–1269.

14 Klein T, Magerl W, Nickel U, Hopf HC, Sandkühler J, Treede RD: Effects of the NMDA-receptor antagonist ketamine on perceptual correlates of long-term potentiation within the nociceptive system. Neuropharmacology 2007;52:655–661.

15 Schulte K, Sollevi A, Segerdahl M: The synergistic effect of combined treatment with systemic ketamine and morphine on experimentally induced windup-like pain in humans. Anesth Analg 2004;98: 1574–1580.

16 Urban MK, Ya Deau JT, Wukovits B, Lipnitsky JY: Ketamine as an adjunct to postoperative pain management in opioid tolerant patients after spinal fusions: a prospective randomized trial. HSS J 2008; 4:62–65.

17 Trujillo KA: The neurobiology of opiate tolerance, dependence and sensitization: mechanisms of NMDA receptor-dependent synaptic plasticity. Neurotox Res 2002;4:373–391.

18 Bell RF, Dahl JB, Moore RA, Kalso E: Perioperative ketamine for acute post-operative pain. Cochrane Database Syst Rev 2006:CD004603.

19 Subramaniam K, Subramaniam B, Steinbrook RA: Ketamine as adjuvant analgesic to opioids: a quantitative and qualitative systematic review. Anesth Analg 2004;99:482–495.

20 Kollender Y, Bickels J, Stocki D, Maruoani N, Chazan S, Nirkin A, Meller I, Weinbroum AA: Subanaesthetic ketamine spares postoperative morphine and controls pain better than standard morphine does alone in orthopaedic-oncological patients. Eur J Cancer 2008;44:954–962.

21 Michelet P, Guervilly C, Hélaine A, Avaro JP, Blayac D, Gaillat F, Dantin T, Thomas P, Kerbaul F: Adding ketamine to morphine for patient-controlled analgesia after thoracic surgery: influence on morphine consumption, respiratory function, and nocturnal desaturation. Br J Anaesth 2007;99:396–403.

22 Cohen SP, Christo PJ, Moroz L: Pain management in trauma patients. Am J Phys Med Rehabil 2004; 83:142–161.

23 Joly V, Richebe P, Guignard B, Fletcher D, Maurette P, Sessler DI, Chauvin M: Remifentanil-induced postoperative hyperalgesia and its prevention with small-dose ketamine. Anesthesiology 2005;103:147–155.

24 Stubhaug A, Breivik H, Eide PK, Kreunen M, Foss A: Mapping of punctuate hyperalgesia around a surgical incision demonstrates that ketamine is a powerful suppressor of central sensitization to pain following surgery. Acta Anaesthesiol Scand 1997;41: 1124–1132.

25 de Kock MF, Lavand'homme PM, Waterloos H: 'Balanced analgesia' in the peri-operative period: is there a place for ketamine? Pain 2001;92:373–380.

26 Engelhardt T, Zaarour C, Naser B, Pehora C, de Ruiter J, Howard A, Crawford MW: Intraoperative low-dose ketamine does not prevent a remifentanil-induced increase in morphine requirement after pediatric scoliosis surgery. Anesth Analg 2008;107: 1170–1175.

27 de Kock M, Lavand'homme PM: The clinical role of NMDA receptor antagonists for the treatment of postoperative pain. Best Pract Res Clin Anaesthesiol 2007;21:85–98.

28 Ayesh EE, Jensen TS, Svensson P: Effects of intra-articular ketamine on pain and somatosensory function in temporomandibular joint arthralgia patients. Pain 2008;137:286–294.

29 Sörensen J, Bengtsson A, Ahlner J, Henriksson KG, Ekselius L, Bengtsson M: Fibromyalgia: are there different mechanisms in the processing of pain? A double blind crossover comparison of analgesic drugs. J Rheumatol 1997;24:1615–1621.

30 Graven-Nielsen T, Aspegren KS, Henriksson KG, Bengtsson M, Sörensen J, Johnson A, Gerdle B, Arendt-Nielsen L: Ketamine reduces muscle pain, temporal summation, and referred pain in fibromyalgia patients. Pain 2000;85:483–491.

31 Wood PB: A reconsideration of the relevance of systemic low-dose ketamine to the pathophysiology of fibromyalgia. J Pain 2006;7:611–614.

32 Carr DB, Goudas LC, Denman WT, Brookoff D, Lavin PT, Staats PS: Safety and efficacy of intranasal ketamine in a mixed population with chronic pain. Pain 2004;110:762–764.

33 Huge V, Lauchart M, Magerl W, Schelling G, Beyer A, Thieme D, Azad SC: Effects of low-dose intranasal (S)-ketamine in patients with neuropathic pain. Eur J Pain 2010;14:387–394.

34 Furuhashi-Yonaha A, Iida H, Asano T, Takeda T, Dohi S: Short- and long-term efficacy of oral ketamine in eight chronic-pain patients. Can J Anaesth 2002;49:886–887.

35 Haines DR, Gaines SP: N of 1 randomised controlled trials of oral ketamine in patients with chronic pain. Pain 1999;83:283–287.

36 Benrath J, Scharbert G, Gustorff B, Adams HA, Kress HG: Long-term intrathecal S(+)-ketamine in a patient with cancer-related neuropathic pain. Br J Anaesth 2005;95:247–249.

37 Muller A, Lemos D: Cancer pain: beneficial effect of ketamine addition to spinal administration of morphine-clonidine-lidocaine mixture. Ann Fr Anesth Reanim 1996;15:271–276.

38 Yang CY, Wong CS, Chang JY, Ho ST: Intrathecal ketamine reduces morphine requirements in patients with terminal cancer pain. Can J Anaesth 1996;43:379–383.

39 Wilson JA, Nimmo AF, Fleetwood-Walker SM, Colvin LA: A randomised double blind trial of the effect of pre-emptive epidural ketamine on persistent pain after lower limb amputation. Pain 2008;135:108–118.

40 Vranken JH, Troost D, Wegener JT, Kruis MR, van der Vegt MH: Neuropathological findings after continuous intrathecal administration of S(+)-ketamine for the management of neuropathic cancer pain. Pain 2005;117:231–235.

41 Cohen SP, Dragovich A: Intrathecal analgesia. Med Clin North Am 2007;91:251–270.

42 Finch PM, Knudsen L, Drummond PD: Reduction of allodynia in patients with complex regional pain syndrome: a double-blind placebo-controlled trial of topical ketamine. Pain 2009;146:18–25.

43 Canbay O, Celebi N, Uzun S, Sahin A, Celiker V, Aypar U: Topical ketamine and morphine for post-tonsillectomy pain. Eur J Anaesthesiol 2008;25:287–292.

44 Murat I, Gall O, Tourniaire B: Procedural pain in children: evidence-based best practices and guidelines. Reg Anesth Pain Med 2003;28:561–572.

45 Lin C, Durieux ME: Ketamine and kids: an update. Ped Anesth 2005;15:91–97.

46 Ramchandra DS, Anisya V, Gourie-Devi M: Ketamine mono-anesthesia for diagnostic muscle biopsy in neuromuscular disorders in infancy and childhood: floppy infant syndrome. Can J Anaesth 1990;37:474–476.

47 Schwartzman RJ, Alexander GM, Grothusen JR, Paylor T, Reichenberger E, Perreault M: Outpatient intravenous ketamine for the treatment of complex regional pain syndrome: a double-blind placebo controlled study. Pain 2009;147:107–115.

48 Goldberg ME, Domsky R, Scaringe D, Hirsh R, Dotson J, Sharaf I, Torjman MC, Schwartzman RJ: Multi-day low dose ketamine infusion for the treatment of complex regional pain syndrome. Pain Physician 2005;8:175–179.

49 Correll GE, Maleki J, Gracely EJ, Muir JJ, Harbut RE: Subanesthetic ketamine infusion therapy: a retrospective analysis of a novel therapeutic approach to complex regional pain syndrome. Pain Med 2004;5:263–275.

50 Eide PK, Stubhaug A, Stenehjem AE: Central dysesthesia pain after traumatic spinal cord injury is dependent on N-methyl-D-aspartate receptor activation. Neurosurgery 1995;37:1080–1087.

51 Kvarnström A, Karlsten R, Quiding H, Gordh T: The analgesic effect of intravenous ketamine and lidocaine on pain after spinal cord injury. Acta Anaesthesiol Scand 2004;48:498–506.

52 Eichenberger U, Neff F, Sveticic G, Björgo S, Petersen-Felix S, Arendt-Nielsen L, Curatolo M: Chronic phantom limb pain: the effects of calcitonin, ketamine, and their combination on pain and sensory thresholds. Anesth Analg 2008;106:1265–1273.

53 Sigtermans MJ, van Hilten JJ, Bauer MC, Arbous MS, Marinus J, Sarton EY, Dahan A: Ketamine produces effective and long-term pain relief in patients with complex regional pain syndrome type 1. Pain 2009;145:304–311.

54 Castrillon EE, Cairns BE, Ernberg M, Wang K, Sessle BJ, Arendt-Nielsen L, Svensson P: Effect of peripheral NMDA receptor blockade with ketamine on chronic myofascial pain in temporomandibular disorder patients: a randomized, double-blinded, placebo-controlled trial. J Orofac Pain 2008;22:122–130.

55 Lemming D, Sörensen J, Graven-Nielsen T, Lauber R, Arendt-Nielsen L, Gerdle B: Managing chronic whiplash associated pain with a combination of low-dose opioid (remifentanil) and NMDA-antagonist (ketamine). Eur J Pain 2007;11:719–732.

56 Gottrup H, Bach FW, Juhl G, Jensen TS: Differential effect of ketamine and lidocaine on spontaneous and mechanical evoked pain in patients with nerve injury pain. Anesthesiology 2006;104:527–536.

Cohen · Liao · Gupta · Plunkett

57 Lynch ME, Clark AJ, Sawynok J, Sullivan MJ: Topical 2% amitriptyline and 1% ketamine in neuropathic pain syndromes: a randomized, double-blind, placebo-controlled trial. Anesthesiology 2005;103:140–146.

58 Jørum E, Warncke T, Stubhaug A: Cold allodynia and hyperalgesia in neuropathic pain: the effect of N-methyl-D-aspartate (NMDA) receptor antagonist ketamine: a double-blind, cross-over comparison with alfentanil and placebo. Pain 2003;101:229–235.

59 Lynch ME, Clark AJ, Sawynok J: A pilot study examining topical amitriptyline, ketamine, and a combination of both in the treatment of neuropathic pain. Clin J Pain 2003;19:323–328.

60 Leung A, Wallace MS, Ridgeway B, Yaksh T: Concentration-effect relationship of intravenous alfentanil and ketamine on peripheral neurosensory thresholds, allodynia and hyperalgesia of neuropathic pain. Pain 2001;91:177–187.

61 Mercadante S, Arcuri E, Tirelli W, Casuccio A: Analgesic effect of intravenous ketamine in cancer patients on morphine therapy: a randomized, controlled, double-blind, crossover, double-dose study. J Pain Symptom Manage 2000;20:246–252.

62 Lauretti GR, Gomes JM, Reis MP, Pereira NL: Low doses of epidural ketamine or neostigmine, but not midazolam, improve morphine analgesia in epidural terminal cancer pain therapy. J Clin Anesth 1999;11:663–668.

63 Rabben T, Skjelbred P, Oye I: Prolonged analgesic effect of ketamine, an N-methyl-D-aspartate receptor inhibitor, in patients with chronic pain. J Pharmacol Exp Ther 1999;289:1060–1066.

64 Persson J, Hasselström J, Wiklund B, Heller A, Svensson JO, Gustafsson LL: The analgesic effect of racemic ketamine in patients with chronic ischemic pain due to lower extremity arteriosclerosis obliterans. Acta Anaesthesiol Scand 1998;42:750–758.

65 Nikolajsen L, Hansen CL, Nielsen J, Keller J, Arendt-Nielsen L, Jensen TS: The effect of ketamine on phantom pain: a central neuropathic disorder maintained by peripheral input. Pain 1996;67:69–77.

66 Felsby S, Nielsen J, Arendt-Nielsen L, Jensen TS: NMDA receptor blockade in chronic neuropathic pain: a comparison of ketamine and magnesium chloride. Pain 1996;64:283–291.

67 Max MB, Byas-Smith MG, Gracely RH, Bennett GJ: Intravenous infusion of the NMDA antagonist, ketamine, in chronic posttraumatic pain with allodynia: a double-blind comparison to alfentanil and placebo. Clin Neuropharmacol 1995;18:360–368.

68 Nicolodi M, Sicuteri F: Exploration of NMDA receptors in migraine: therapeutic and theoretic implications. Int J Clin Pharmacol Res 1995;15:181–189.

69 Eide PK, Jørum E, Stubhaug A, Bremnes J, Breivik H: Relief of post-herpetic neuralgia with the N-methyl-D-aspartic acid receptor antagonist ketamine: a double-blind, cross-over comparison with morphine and placebo. Pain 1994;58:347–354.

70 Backonja M, Arndt G, Gombar KA, Check B, Zimmermann M: Response of chronic neuropathic pain syndromes to ketamine: a preliminary study. Pain 1994;56:51–57.

71 Ryan AJ, Lin F, Atayee RS: Ketamine mouthwash for mucositis pain. J Palliat Med 2009;12:989–991.

72 Kiefer RT, Rohr P, Ploppa A, Dieterich HJ, Grothusen J, Koffler S, Altemeyer KH, Unertl K, Schwartzman RJ: Efficacy of ketamine in anesthetic dosage for the treatment of refractory complex regional pain syndrome: an open-label phase II study. Pain Med 2008;9:1173–1201.

73 Finkel JC, Pestieau SR, Quezado ZM: Ketamine as an adjuvant for treatment of cancer pain in children and adolescents. J Pain 2007;8:515–521.

74 Webster LR, Walker MJ: Safety and efficacy of prolonged outpatient ketamine infusions for neuropathic pain. Am J Ther 2006;13:300–305.

75 Kannan TR, Saxena A, Bhatnagar S, Barry A: Oral ketamine as an adjuvant to oral morphine for neuropathic pain in cancer patients. J Pain Symptom Manage 2002;23:60–65.

76 Kiefer RT, Rohr P, Unertl K, Altmeyer KH, Grothusen J, Schwartzman RJ: Recovery from intractable complex regional pain syndrome type-I (RSD) under high dose intravenous ketamine-midazolam sedation. Neurology 2002;58:A474.

77 Jackson K, Ashby M, Martin P, Pisasale M, Brumley D, Hayes B: 'Burst' ketamine for refractory cancer pain: an open-label audit of 39 patients. J Pain Symptom Manage 2002;22:834–842.

78 Lauretti GR, Lima IC, Reis MP, Prado WA, Pereira NL: Oral ketamine and transdermal nitroglycerin as analgesic adjuvants to oral morphine therapy for cancer pain management. Anesthesiology 1999;90:1528–1533.

79 Grape S, Tramèr MR: Do we need preemptive analgesia for the treatment of postoperative pain? Best Pract Res Clin Anaesthesiol 2007;21:51–63.

80 Burton AW, Lee DH, Saab C, Chung JM: Preemptive intrathecal ketamine injection produces a long-lasting decrease in neuropathic pain behavior in a rat model. Reg Anesth Pain Med 1999;24:208–213.

81 Buvanendran A, Kroin JS: Useful adjuvants for postoperative pain management. Best Pract Res Clin Anaesthesiol 2007;21:31–49.

82 Ong CK, Lirk P, Seymour RA, Jenkins BJ: The efficacy of preemptive analgesia for acute postoperative pain management: a meta-analysis. Anesth Analg 2005;100:754–773.

83 O'Flaherty JE, Lin CX: Does ketamine or magnesium affect posttonsillectomy pain in children? Paediatr Anaesth 2003;13:413–421.

84 Köknel Talu G, Ozyalçın NS, Balsak R, Karadeniz M: The efficacy of preemptive ketamine and ropivacaine in pediatric patients: a placebo controlled, double-blind study (in Turkish). Agri 2008;20:31–36.

85 Becke K, Albrecht S, Schmitz B, Rech D, Koppert W, Schüttler J, Hering W: Intraoperative low-dose S-ketamine has no preventive effects on postoperative pain and morphine consumption after major urological surgery in children. Paediatr Anaesth 2005;15:484–490.

86 Kim HY, Yoon HS: The effects of ketamine preemptive analgesia on postoperative pain in patients undergoing a hysterectomy (in Korean). Taehan Kanho Hakhoe Chi 2006;36:114–126.

87 Lebrun T, van Elstraete AC, Sandefo I, Polin B, Pierre-Louis L: Lack of a pre-emptive effect of low-dose ketamine on post-operative pain following oral surgery. Can J Anaesth 2006;53:146–152.

88 Katz J, Schmid R, Snijdelaar DG, Coderre TJ, McCartney CJ, Wowk A: Pre-emptive analgesia using intravenous fentanyl plus low-dose ketamine for radical prostatectomy under general anesthesia does not produce short-term or long-term reductions in pain or analgesic use. Pain 2004;110:707–718.

89 Woolf CJ: Pain: moving from symptom control toward mechanism-specific pharmacologic management. Ann Intern Med 2004;140:441–451.

90 Graven-Nielsen T, Aspegren KS, Henriksson KG, Bengtsson M, Sörensen J, Johnson A, Gerdle B, Arendt-Nielsen L: Ketamine reduces muscle pain, temporal summation, and referred pain in fibromyalgia patients. Pain 2000;85:483–491.

91 Sörensen J, Bengtsson A, Bäckman E, Henriksson KG, Bengtsson M: Pain analysis in patients with fibromyalgia: effects of intravenous morphine, lidocaine, and ketamine. Scand J Rheumatol 1995;24:360–365.

92 Guedj E, Cammilleri S, Colavolpe C, de Laforte C, Niboyet J, Mundler O: Follow-up of pain processing recovery after ketamine in hyperalgesic fibromyalgia patients using brain perfusion ECD-SPECT. Eur J Nucl Med Mol Imaging 2007;34:2115–2119.

93 Cohen SP, Chang AS, Larkin T, Mao J: The IV ketamine test: a predictive response tool for an oral dextromethorphan treatment regimen in neuropathic pain. Anesth Analg 2004;99:1753–1759.

94 Cohen SP, Verdolin MH, Chang AS, Kurihara C, Morlando BJ, Mao J: The IV ketamine test predicts subsequent response to an oral dextromethorphan treatment regimen in fibromyalgia patients. J Pain 2006;7:391–398.

95 Cohen SP, Wang S, Chen L, Kurihara C, McKnight G, Marcuson M, Mao J: An intravenous ketamine test as a predictive response tool in opioid-exposed patients with persistent pain. J Pain Symptom Manage 2009;37:698–708.

96 Cohen SP, Kapoor S, Rathmell JP: Intravenous infusions tests have limited utility for selecting long-term drug therapy in patients with chronic pain: a systematic review. Anesthesiology 2009;111:416–431.

97 Green SM, Krauss B: Clinical practice guideline for emergency department ketamine dissociative sedation in children. Ann Emerg Med 2004;44:460–471.

98 Morgan CJ, Curran HV: Acute and chronic effects of ketamine upon human memory: a review. Psychopharmacology (Berl) 2006;188:408–424.

99 Morgan CJ, Monaghan L, Curran HV: Beyond the K-hole: a 3-year longitudinal investigation of the cognitive and subjective effects of ketamine in recreational users who have substantially reduced their use of the drug. Addiction 2004;99:1450–1461.

100 Olney J, Labruyère J, Wang G, Wozniak DF, Price MT, Sesma MA: NMDA antagonist neurotoxicity: mechanism and prevention. Science 1991;254:1515–1518.

101 Bernstein HG, Becker A, Keilhoff G, Spilker C, Gorczyca WA, Braunewell KH, Grecksch G: Brain region-specific changes in the expression of calcium sensor proteins after repeated applications of ketamine to rats. Neurosci Lett 2003;339:95–98.

102 Keilhoff G, Becker A, Grecksch G, Wolf G, Bernstein HG: Repeated application of ketamine to rats induces changes in the hippocampal expression of parvalbumin, neuronal nitric oxide synthase and cFOS similar to those found in human schizophrenia. Neuroscience 2004;126:591–598.

103 Olney JW, Labruyère J, Price MT: Pathological changes induced in cerebrocortical neurons by phencyclidine and related drugs. Science 1989;244:1360–1362.

104 Hayashi H, Dikkes P, Soriano SG: Repeated administration of ketamine may lead to neuronal degeneration in the developing rat brain. Paediatr Anesth 2002;12:770–774.

105 Ikonomidou C, Bosch F, Miksa M, Bittigau P, Vöckler J, Dikranian K, Tenkova TI, Stefovska V, Turski L, Olney JW: Blockade of the NMDA receptors and apoptotic neurodegeneration in the developing brain. Science 1999;283:70–74.

106 Young C, Jevtovic-Todorovic V, Qin YQ, Tenkova T, Wang H, Labruyère J, Olney JW: Potential of ketamine and midazolam, individually or in combination, to induce apoptotic neurodegeneration in the infant mouse brain. Br J Pharmacol 2005;146:189–197.

107 Slikker W Jr, Zou X, Hotchkiss CE, Divine RL, Sadovova N, Twaddle NC, Doerge DR, Scallet AC, Patterson TA, Hanig JP, Paule MG, Wang C: Ketamine-induced neuronal cell death in the perinatal rhesus monkey. Toxicol Sci 2007;98:145–158.

108 Zou X, Patterson TA, Divine RL, Sadovova N, Zhang X, Hanig JP, Paule MG, Slikker W Jr, Wang C: Prolonged exposure to ketamine increases neurodegeneration in the developing monkey brain. Int J Dev Neurosci 2009;27:727–731.

109 Vutskits L, Gascon E, Potter G, Tassonyi E, Kiss JZ: Low concentrations of ketamine initiate dendritic atrophy of differentiated GABAergic neurons in culture. Toxicology 2007;234:216–226.

110 Church J, Zeman S, Lodge D: The neuroprotective action of ketamine and MK-801 after transient cerebral ischemia in rats. Anesthesiology 1988;69: 702–709.

111 Shapira Y, Artru AA, Lam AM: Ketamine decreases cerebral infarct volume and improves neurological outcome following experimental head trauma in rats. J Neurosurg Anesthesiol 1992;4:231–240.

112 Shapira Y, Lam AM, Eng CC, Laohaprasit V, Michel M: Therapeutic time window and dose response of the beneficial effects of ketamine in experimental head injury. Stroke 1994;25:1637–1643.

113 Spandou E, Karkavelas G, Soubasi V, Avgovstides-Savvopoulou P, Loizidis T, Guiba-Tziampiri O: Effect of ketamine on hypoxic-ischemic brain damage in newborn rats. Brain Res 1999;819:1–7.

114 Anand KJ, Garg S, Rovnaghi CR, Narsinghani U, Bhutta AT, Hall RW: Ketamine reduces the cell death following inflammatory pain in newborn rat brain. Pediatr Res 2007;62:283–290.

115 Petersen RC, Stillman RC: Phencyclidine: an overview. NIDA Res Monogr 1978;21:1–17.

116 Murphy R, Roe S: Drug misuse declared: findings from the 2006/2007 British Crime Survey. London, Home Office Research, Development and Statistics Directorate, 2007.

117 Muetzelfeldt L, Kamboj SK, Rees H, Taylor J, Morgan CJ, Curran HV: Journey through the K-hole: phenomenological aspects of ketamine use. Drug Alcohol Depend 2008;95:219–229.

118 Zhuo X, Cang Y, Yan H, Bu J, Shen B: The prevalence of drugs in motor vehicle accidents and traffic violations in Shanghai and neighboring cities. Accid Anal Prev 2010;42:2179–2184.

119 Wong OF, Tsui KL, Lam TS, Sze NN, Wong SC, Lau FL, Liu SH: Prevalence of drugged drivers among non-fatal driver casualties presenting to a trauma centre in Hong Kong. Hong Kong Med J 2010;16: 246–251.

120 Cheng JY, Chan DT, Mok VK: An epidemiological study on alcohol/drugs related fatal traffic crash cases of deceased drivers in Hong Kong between 1996 and 2000. Forensic Sci Int 2005;153: 196–201.

Steven P. Cohen, MD
Johns Hopkins Pain Management Division
550 North Broadway, Suite 301
Baltimore, MD 21029 (USA)
Tel. +1 410 955 1818, E-Mail scohen40@jhmi.edu

Subject Index